SEVEN STEPS to STOP a HEART ATTACK

DR. BOB ARNOT

Simon & Schuster Paperbacks
New York London Toronto Sydney

SIMON & SCHUSTER PAPERBACKS
Rockefeller Center
1230 Avenue of the Americas
New York, NY 10020

Copyright © 2005 by Dr. Bob Arnot
Illustrations copyright © 2005 by medmovie.com
All rights reserved,
including the right of reproduction
in whole or in part in any form.

First Simon & Schuster paperback edition 2006

SIMON & SCHUSTER and colophon are registered trademarks
of Simon & Schuster, Inc.

For information about special discounts for bulk purchases,
please contact Simon & Schuster Special Sales at
1-800-456-6798 or business@simonandschuster.com.

Designed by Karolina Harris

Manufactured in the United States of America

10   9   8   7   6   5   4   3   2   1

The Library of Congress has catalogued the hardcover edition as follows:
Arnot, Robert Burns.
    Seven steps to stop a heart attack / Bob Arnot.
        p. cm.
    Includes index.
1. Coronary heart disease—Popular works. I. Title.
RC685.C6A76 2005
616.1'2305—dc22   2004052484

ISBN-13: 978-0-7432-2557-1
ISBN-10:   0-7432-2557-0
ISBN-13: 978-0-7432-2559-5 (Pbk)
ISBN-10:   0-7432-2559-7 (Pbk)

This publication contains the opinions and ideas of its author. It is intended to provide helpful and informative material on the subjects addressed in the publication. It is sold with the understanding that the author and publisher are not engaged in rendering medical, health, or any other kind of personal professional services in the book. The reader should consult his or her medical, health, or other competent professional before adopting any of the suggestions in this book or drawing inferences from it.

The author and publisher specifically disclaim all responsibility for any liability, loss, or risk, personal or otherwise, which is incurred as a consequence, directly or indirectly, of the use and application of any of the contents of this book.

*This book is dedicated
to my beloved father,
whose tragic death from heart disease
inspired me to write this book . . .*

*And to Dr. Reed Quinn and
the magnificent physicians, nurses,
and staff of the Maine Medical Center
who saved my mother's life.*

ACKNOWLEDGMENTS

GEOFF Kloske: Geoff was the perfect editor, incisive and skillful. He always had fresh and inspiring ideas on how to make this book even better. I'll always be grateful to Geoff for the compassion he showed when my father died suddenly from a heart attack. I'll never forget his understanding and help.

David Rosenthal: Special thanks to David Rosenthal, my publisher, for having the vision to make *Seven Steps to Stop a Heart Attack* happen and for putting such an outstanding team behind it. I prize David for his unending enthusiasm and great good nature, which were sources of wonderful inspiration.

Suzanne C. Bagin: My associate in writing this book, Suzanne showed ceaseless energy and amazing attention to detail. Her inquisitive mind and investigative skills brought a treasure trove of wonderful material to this book. Suzanne's ability to work tirelessly kept this book on track and on schedule.

Dan and Simon Green: To my indefatigable agents who've always been there for me, for their hard work and devotion.

CONTENTS

Contents

PREFACE

In a small village in northern Italy called Limone sul Garda live people with astonishingly little heart disease. Their bodies produce a protein called ApoA-I Milano. This protein appears to be as close to a miracle substance as has even been found in the century-long history of modern cardiology. ApoA-I Milano strikes at the epicenter of heart disease, the soft fatty core of the blockages found in coronary arteries. ApoA-I Milano rapidly mobilizes cholesterol and transports it away, sharply decreasing the size of the blockage. What truly blows researchers away is how quickly ApoA-I Milano works.

The conventional wisdom is that it takes many years of rigorous dieting, exercise, and medications even to begin to make a dent in lowering cholesterol. Yet ApoA-I works in as little as forty-eight hours!

This has completely revolutionized the thinking of cardiologists like the Cleveland Clinic's Dr. Steven Nissen, who now sees coronary artery disease as a tremendously dynamic condition capable of breathtaking changes in very short periods of time.

Just five weekly treatments of ApoA-I Milano, called ETC-216 in its pharmaceutical form, in human beings produced significant regression of coronary artery disease. ApoA-I has been used alone, but already cardiologists are planning to use it with other lifesaving medications such as statins. The future of heart disease therapy may look like that of certain cancers cures—a cocktail of drugs, each hitting a different target. The up-and-coming heart disease cocktails will cure the disease, say many of the nation's top cardiologists, entirely preventing heart attacks and deaths from heart disease in much of the population—if begun early enough.

New miracle drugs are even more critical to immediate lifesaving efforts. Doctors used to think of coronary artery disease as discrete blockages in the arteries that could be easily seen on coronary angiograms and treated with surgery or balloon therapy. Now a new research device called intravascular ultrasound paints a much more alarming picture. While a single large blockage may be visible on an angiogram, there may be dozens of submerged plaques that show only as small blockages or don't show at all. The ultrasound shows that the submerged plaques are *huge*. In effect, it's like having the street in front of your house lined with dozens of improvised explosive devices, mines and grenades, any one of which could explode at any moment. You may see one at the end of your driveway, but all the rest are buried.

The smartest strategy is to defuse these explosive devices. Diffusing an entire artery can be done only with medication or by completely bypassing it. Fortunately, as you'll read in the chapter on medications, this can be done quickly and effectively.

The most stunning development in the long history of cardiology may be the breathtaking new miracle drugs that can save your life in *weeks*. That's the good news. The bad news is that the vast majority of Americans with heart disease are not following even the most basic course of action—with tragic results.

Many of us need a highly customized treatment program, but few receive it. It's a lesson I learned the hard way, in the case of my own father, who died suddenly, tragically, and unexpectedly before I researched and wrote this book.

This book will help you become a smart consumer, able to navigate the treacherous shoals of modern cardiology, whether you are at low, moderate, or high risk.

It works. Using the exact steps in this book, my mother's life was miraculously saved when heart disease came within minutes of killing her.

INTRODUCTION

THE late winter morning broke with bright blue skies, a stiff breeze, and mild temperatures. The top of Stowe, Vermont's Mount Mansfield reappeared from the mists for the first time after several days of snow. Freshly groomed ski slopes invited early skiers to a smooth, fast run. In line for the high-speed quad lift, I looked down at my cell phone's LCD panel. It showed a missed call from my parents' home outside Boston. I returned the call, which was answered by my nephew Mathew, a graduate student at MIT.

"Something's wrong with your father," Mathew told me. A million thoughts raced through my mind. I knew my father had heart problems. How quickly could I be at my father's side? Is he getting the right care? Can I get through to the doctor in the emergency room? Are there special techniques he's not getting that he should? Should they rush him into surgery? Should he have clot-busting drugs? How could I make all this happen quickly enough to save his life? None of it was necessary. "He's dead," my nephew said.

Those chilling words heralded the end of the life of one of the people I most loved in this world. I couldn't believe it. The words kept echoing through my head. Just the night before, he'd asked for help with his health. Just days earlier, he had told his personal trainer he wanted to walk again without a cane. I was so eager to help, and now there was nothing I could ever do. I was powerless. For you, however, it is not too late. You still have the power to save your life or that of someone you love.

Ironically, my father's cardiologist had told him he'd never die of a heart attack. Every time I asked my father why he refused to consider further testing or more therapy, he repeated his doctor's reassurance. Yet his life ended due to a sudden and massive cardiovascular event, complete with the classic warning signs of a heart attack in an older patient (you'll learn these in Step 2, "Know the Warning Signs"). I'd watched dozens of men die in emergency rooms because they had waited too long and ignored their symptoms. My father's symptoms had increased for days. But reassured by his cardiologist's words of comfort, he never sought help, never called his doctor. I had asked him to get a stress test, but he insisted it wasn't necessary. I'd pleaded with his cardiologist to put him on a few key lifesaving medications. The cardiologist said he would take it up with my father's primary care doctor. Whether the primary care doctor failed to convince my father or opted not to prescribe the medicine I recommended, we will never know. Even after one cardiologist told my father that he had suffered damage to his heart, and I recommended stress testing, I was never able to ascertain that any of the testing was done. Of course, my father, like many patients, was resistant to taking new medication, and from time to time even advised his doctors not to talk to me, since he believed his health care was his own business.

Tragedies like my father's are repeated hundreds of times every day across America. The information and technology are there to save lives, but patients fail to receive the care they need or deserve. Much of what they need is cheap and easily available, emphasizes Dr. Claude Lenfant, former longtime director of the National Heart, Lung, and Blood Institute (NHLBI). Yet despite years of talking prevention, too few doctors ever come through. High-tech lifesaving techniques also make a big difference, but too few Americans know how or when to access them, or fail to get them done properly. The simple and frightening fact is that the vast majority of Americans do not get state-of-the-art treatment for their heart disease, at a cost of hundreds of thousands of lives every year.

This isn't just my observation but also that of the country's best cardiologists. Take Cornell's Dr. Jeffrey Borer. "It does seem that the average person isn't always getting the appropriate diagnostic tests, the most effective preventive strategies, and the most useful treatments. The reasons are not absolutely clear, but the situation may result in part from the increasing explosion of medical knowledge, with the need for greater and greater specialization by practitioners in order to remain at the cutting edge in a particular area. The result may be a mismatch between the patient's problem and the expertise of the doctor he or she has approached for evaluation and help. It's important to know what you don't know, as well as what you know, in order to provide optimal advice to a patient and to seek additional help when needed."

Other physicians, such as Dr. Claude Lenfant, believe that's being kind. How could so few patients receive the proper care when we know that heart disease is the number one cause of death in America and quickly heading to the top of the list in dozens of countries around the world? Wouldn't all doctors have the same routine standard of care? What is it that Americans are missing in preventing, detecting, and treating heart disease? As was the case with my father, there is a cascade of measures that start from the most basic prevention. How bad is this failure to diagnose and treat properly?

Massive. Coronary artery disease is preventable. Coronary artery disease is potentially reversible. How then can 700,000 Americans die each year of a heart attack, according to the latest American Heart Association data? How can half of them die without ever reaching a hospital bed?

I'm not talking about the slow ebbing of life due to heart failure. Most often death is a sudden, catastrophic event, which should be preventable given the huge wealth of new information, new medications, and cutting-edge technologies. Throughout this book I look for the missing half, the half of all heart patients who slip through the system only to suffer a heart attack or die suddenly and seemingly without warning—just like my father. In researching this book I found that doctors rarely talked about the missing half. There is no great effort to find or treat these patients before they suffer a heart attack or die, undetected in advance by the medical system. It's become just an acceptable part of doing business. Finding this silent majority would save more lives than curing cancer and AIDS combined! Relative to AIDS and cancer, these are *easy* saves.

In addition to the missing half, there are those who have heart attacks and, unbelievably, don't know it. These are purely silent heart attacks. According to the famous Framingham study, the oldest, longest, biggest, and most important of all studies examining the epidemiology of heart disease, 28 percent of men and 33 percent of women were found to have had heart attacks only on a routine visit to their doctor, months or years after the attack. Here are the details. Patients were undergoing EKGs every two years. Doctors noticed definite evidence of heart attacks on the EKGs. (An EKG is an electrical tracing on a piece of paper, which can show distinctive markings of a heart attack, such as a deep depression called a Q wave.) When doctors interviewed these patients, they found about one-third were never hospitalized for the heart attack. They also found that these men and women had nothing that sounded like a heart attack in the two years between the time the EKG was normal and the time it became abnormal.

The prestigious Centers for Disease Control (CDC) estimates that each year 400,000 to 460,000 people die from heart disease in an emergency department or before reaching a hospital, which accounts for more than 60 percent of all cardiac deaths. Who missed the boat? Who forgot to check their complete cholesterol screen? Who forgot to take a complete history? Who forgot to call 911? Who forgot to lower their cholesterol or blood pressure to the proper level? Who forgot to educate these patients about unusual symptoms? It just boggles the mind. That degree of failure is unheard of in virtually any other arena. Imagine if half of airplanes weren't inspected and maintained and half of them eventually crashed. No one would fly. I make the case through this book that, like my father, the vast majority of these heart attacks and deaths are unforced errors by health care providers and patients. Pure and simple, most could be prevented. In no other area of medicine, in no other walk of life, is the rate of failure as high or catastrophic.

My own mother was allowed to deteriorate into congestive heart failure and near death by a top Harvard doctor, when she should have had a standard cardiogram and been referred to a surgeon.

There are huge variations in medical practice. Even though the standard of care may be well laid out in medical literature, your chance of receiving that standard of excellence is small. The average hospital stay for heart disease has been shortened, as measured in the current Medicare data. This means that there is a limited opportunity for the health care team to counsel patients about diet, exercise, and smoking cessation after a first heart attack to prevent a second one. Simply put, the implementation of risk-reducing strategies is poor. Doctors like myself pull their hair out, knowing how amazing the power of prevention is, only to see so many bodies washed under the bridge due to lack of delivery. Let's look at more evidence.

A Duke University study that found hospitals that did not follow treatment guidelines put heart attack patients at a one-third greater risk of dying before discharge compared to patients treated at hospitals that did comply with recommended guidelines. What was the chance of getting the right treatment, according to the guidelines? Astonishingly, this study found that close to 300 hospitals did not always comply with the recommended care, from clot-busting drugs to lifesaving balloon therapy. Only 40 percent of patients with congestive heart failure got the life-extending ACE inhibitors at what were considered the leading hospitals. Thirty percent of those same hospitals failed to give the right drugs.

The story is even worse for women. More women than men now die of heart disease. A study of 2,763 postmenopausal women with heart disease found that doctors failed to prescribe even the most basic preventive medicines, including aspirin, beta-blockers, and cholesterol-lowering drugs. Why? Some doctors still see heart disease as a predominantly male disease even though it is the number one killer of women. One famous slogan, obscure in origin, is echoed by researchers in women's heart disease at leading institutions: "Show me a man with chest pain and I'll show you a heart attack. Show me a woman with chest pain and I'll show you anxiety." My poor mother had the classic signs of congestive heart failure, yet she told me that her Harvard doctor told her there was no change in her condition and to return in six months!

The American Heart Association journal *Circulation* reported in 2003 that "most women who die from cardiac death have no prior history of heart disease. However, 94 percent of these women have at least one cardiac risk factor such as smoking, high blood pressure, high cholesterol, diabetes or obesity." Dr. Christine Albert of Brigham and Women's Hospital in Boston says the concern is that doctors tend to focus on preventing sudden cardiac death in patients with documented heart disease but not those with risk factors only. One of my closest friends died suddenly just one day after seeing her cardiologist, where she complained of symptoms of increasingly severe heart disease.

The worst record is found for patients with high blood pressure. Only half of America's 50 million hypertensives are treated with drugs at all. In only a quarter is blood pressure adequately controlled and even less in older or black patients. High blood pressure is one of the earliest identifiable risk factors for heart disease.

Dr. Claude Lenfant says that statins may be the biggest life-saving revolution in cardiology, but only a minority of those who should be on these cholesterol-lowering drugs are. Here are the statistics for patients with high cholesterol: 60 percent (that's almost two-thirds!) are totally unaware that their cholesterol is high. Worse, only 14.5 percent take cholesterol-lowering medication, and a mere 6.5 percent succeed in lowering their cholesterol to the recommended range.

Even the vice president of the United States, Dick Cheney, prior to his fourth heart attack, was not receiving the state-of-the-art care that top cardiologists at institutions like the Cleveland Clinic believe he should have had.

To summarize, the extent of this tragedy is almost beyond comprehension. Here you have the number one killer in the United States, yet for half of its victims, sudden death is their first evidence of heart disease. Dr. Joseph Ornato, professor and chairman of the Department of Emergency Medicine at Virginia Commonwealth University/Medical College of Virginia, points out that only about 4 to 6 percent of these sudden deaths are true heart attacks with classic symptoms. This means that 94 to 96 percent of them simply drop dead with no warning. That's a frightening number.

As doctors, we have gotten so complacent about these statistics that they have become background noise. It took the death of my father to bring home the terrible impact that each individual loss makes. It took my mother's near death to make me believe a few basic steps can save lives.

This book contains everything you need to know to save your life from heart disease. Heart disease is still the disease most likely to kill you, yet amazing technological marvels can radically improve your quality of life and keep you alive years longer. The trouble is that the highly specialized knowledge is deeply fragmented. One of my father's physicians, a world-renowned expert in one facet of noninvasive cardiology, failed, in my view (and I'm sure he'd disagree), to deliver state-of-the-art preventive care for coronary artery disease or congestive heart failure. In all fairness, my father may have resisted taking any more medications, and his doctors may have failed to convince him of the necessity of such medications.

Regardless of the explanation, it is still my view that my father did not receive state-of-the-art preventive care. This is upsetting, but I promise you that the rest of this book solves problems. The good news about heart disease is nothing less than amazing for those who seek and receive excellence. Dr. Paul Ridker, director of the Center for Cardiovascular Disease Prevention at Brigham and Women's Hospital, says, "This is a phenomenally interesting period of time. What we know now about heart disease is just extraordinary compared to what we knew eight to nine years ago. We literally are sitting in the middle of a revolution in our understanding of what causes this plaque in the heart's arteries and what causes these plaques to rupture and cause a heart attack." In the blizzard of daily health reports on TV and radio and in the newspapers, the big picture has obscured the dramatic, near-miraculous advances that have been made in the prevention and treatment of heart disease.

Of all the major killers in the world, coronary artery disease is the best to have. Why? It's the number one killer in America, it's terribly incapacitating, and you can die suddenly and catastrophically. Am I crazy? Not at all. Cancer, diabetes, obesity, Parkinson's disease, HIV—I'd take heart disease over any of them. Of all the major killers, heart disease is the one that you can walk away from. It's the one disease with which you can live a completely normal and long life. It's the one disease that is actually reversible. Too few Americans ever get to avail themselves of these opportunities and end up paying with their lives.

I wrote this book so that you and members of your family won't have to suffer the awful fate that awaited my father. Much of what you'll read here is new and even surprising. You may have caught snippets of new "breakthroughs" on the evening news but don't know how these might apply to you. Virtually no one I know, including very good doctors and even cardiologists, has the big picture. One doctor may put you on a lifesaving drug only to miss a key diagnostic test. Another doctor may know where to refer you but miss your symptoms. This book will put you in the driver's seat with the big picture, so you can put together a comprehensive program that *will* save your life. Do you have a ticking time bomb in your chest? Chances are you do. The only question is, how long is the fuse? Will it explode fifteen years from now, or fifteen minutes.

THE GOOD NEWS

The black suburban battlewagon drove deliberately up to George Washington Medical Center emergency room entrance. Men in dark suits and sunglasses, talking into their wrist radios, formed a protective cordon. Dick Cheney, vice president of the United States, walked in under his own steam, observed closely by the Secret Service. Word leaked out that he had suffered a heart attack. This would be number four, a disaster for most people. But with leading-edge new therapy, Dick Cheney was back at work within days—nothing short of a miracle. A 90 percent blockage was found in one of his coronary arteries. His cardiologist pushed aside the blockage with a balloon at the end of a long catheter and a inserted a stent to keep his artery open and prevent any further damage. Forty-six years earlier, when President Eisenhower had his heart attack, there was little doctors could do but put him to bed for weeks. Fifty-seven years earlier, Franklin Roosevelt died with his blood pressure wildly out of control. There was nothing Roosevelt's doctor could do.

There has been a revolution in cardiology over the last five years, and American lives are being saved by the tens of thousands.

Conventional wisdom: High technology can pull me from the jaws of death.
The real deal: Not if you don't get there on time.

The good news is embodied in one man, Dick Cheney. Remarkably, here's a man with four heart attacks, a potential human wreck who managed to become and serve as vice president of the United States. His disease was premature, beginning in his forties. He had undergone angioplasty several times and a bypass-grafting procedure. He developed an electrophysiological abnormality that could have killed him in a second. If he died tomorrow, his care would still be a major triumph, preserving more than two decades of useful life. By jumping into action at the earliest sign of trouble, he succeeded, beyond most cardiologists' wildest imaginations. Ten years ago, the possibility of his very survival would have been questionable. The great good news is that, if you know what to do, you can live years, even decades longer than if you don't, even if you're not the vice president.

Heart attacks used to kill us in our forties and fifties. When I was in medical school, I saw coronary care units full of men in the prime of their lives. "That death rate is so low now that we're no longer able to track it. It's almost gone," Dr. Teri Manolio, director of the epidemiology and biometry programs at the National Heart, Lung, and Blood Institute, told Gina Kolata of *The New York Times*. Huge strides have been made in treating coronary artery disease. Now most patients who are dying of heart disease are men and women in their seventies and eighties. Amazing technological and conceptual breakthroughs have made this possible. This book will let you take advantage of these with the object of preventing heart disease, so you can live healthy to a very old age. Claude Lenfant adds, "In the old days, you had a heart attack and you died. You were almost signing the death certificate in advance. Now you know you can get another twenty or maybe twenty-five years," he told *The New York Times*. But even though you're less likely to die early, you're more likely to have heart disease. By 2050, the number of people with heart disease will *double*.

All this should give you great hope. No matter how severe your heart disease is, or how big your risk of potential catastrophe is, you could have a bright and long future ahead. Heart disease begins when you are young but first shows up in middle age. One in six teenagers autopsied after fatal car crashes already had large plaques in his or her coronary arteries. One in three teenagers have buildups by age thirty, and 50 percent of people over thirty have them. In your fifties, it's an astounding 85 percent. Heart disease is progressive. In nearly every one of us, year by year, the disease is growing in our arteries. The great news is that you can stop that disease now.

In Step 6, "Take Lifesaving Medications," I look at how medical therapy alone can actually slow or stop the progression of coronary artery disease and can extend your life by years. In Step 7, "Get the Right Lifesaving Procedure," I look at how to stop a heart attack cold with balloon therapy and how to keep arteries open for years to decades with breakthrough stents that contain drugs that prevent new blockages. I also look at clot-busting drugs and other medications used during a heart attack.

STEP ONE: KNOW THE ENEMIES

THERE is a revolution in heart disease, blowing away decades of misconceptions about the root cause of heart attacks and therefore how they should best be treated. In this step I look at the enemies. The first part, on fracture, lays out the most up-to-date and revolutionary understanding of heart attacks. The second part, on inflammation, explores the most recently discovered cause of heart attacks. And the third part, on the accelerator, looks at how even the mildest elevations in blood sugar can lead to the rapid and fatal acceleration of heart disease in a condition with the sinister name of metabolic syndrome.

FRACTURE

The emergency room at the old Peter Bent Brigham Hospital in Boston was as rough-and-tumble as they got. Its appearance was pure inner city—jammed to overflowing with deathly ill and injured patients, gurneys flying through the hallways, sleep-starved interns on their last legs, blood techs rushing fresh units of plasma into surgery. Amid this apparent chaos arrived a slightly balding businessman in his early fifties, lying on an ambulance stretcher and appearing terrified. His forehead was cool to the touch yet he was drenched with sweat. He complained of a deep aching pain in his chest and pain down his left arm and into his back. A member of the clinical staff slid his EKG between his fingers, reading it as it came off the machine as if it were a stock tickertape. The doctor looked over the top of his bifocals and said impassionedly, "You're having a very serious heart attack."

Conventional wisdom: I know all about heart disease.
The real deal: Don't overlook the obvious.

This man had every major symptom of a classic heart attack. He also had every major risk factor. I was a medical student at the time. The doctor turned to me and said, "Smoker. We don't usually see heart attacks at this age unless they smoke." He had elevated cholesterol, high blood pressure, and strong family history. He'd also never seen a cardiologist.

In this book I look at fascinating new discoveries that explain the previously unexplainable—why patients without known risk factors or with weak risk factors have heart attacks and die. Still, I don't want to take your focus off the obvious, the classic heart attack with the classic risk factors. You can be every bit as dead with plain vanilla high cholesterol as with the exotic newly uncovered risks—inflammation and metabolic syndrome. These new risks may explain why many people without classic risk factors still have heart disease and die.

What's changed since I was a medical student is our understanding of what causes the classic heart attack: the sudden and precipitous fracture of a plaque in the coronary artery. This realization changes how heart disease is best prevented and treated, even in its most classic form.

Classic theory still holds that cholesterol is deposited in the walls of your coronary arteries, beginning as early as grade school. Over the years, these plaques grow larger and larger. These are still the basics, and that's where classic risk factors come in. If you have these—high cholesterol, smoking, elevated blood pressure—there's an excellent chance that you are laying down the foundations for a heart attack in your future.

CLASSIC RISK FACTORS

The longest and most important study in the history of heart disease began in late 1948 in Framingham, Massachusetts, virtually next door to the town I grew up in. Framingham was picked because its families tended to stay there generation after generation, making it much easier for researchers to keep track of succeeding generations. Each subject underwent a comprehensive history and physical exam. With great foresight, the researchers took blood samples and froze the serum for the future. If they didn't know what to look for then, they could always look back decades later.

After twenty years, data showed that heart attacks and death from heart disease occurred among people with three key risks: smoking, high blood pressure, and high total cholesterol. As the years went by, the findings got more specific, discovering that the cholesterol measurement required more sophistication: teasing out "good" cholesterol from "bad." The Greenland study confirms the importance of these risk factors, reporting that as many as 85 percent of patients suffering heart attacks have at least one classic risk factor.

CLASSIC CORONARY ARTERY DISEASE

In the testing and treatment chapters of this book, I look at the rationale for specific tests, drugs, procedures, and surgeries. In the brief description of classic coronary artery disease below, you'll gain a solid understanding of the underlying principles of those treatments. I firmly believe that understanding the disease will strongly motivate you to select a far more comprehensive treatment program. Without this understanding, you may not buy the rationale for taking statins, aspirin, ACE inhibitors, beta-blockers, and other key medications that may well save your life. For instance, my mother asked me, "I'm taking aspirin, why would I have to take a statin?" As you'll see, statins and aspirin work in completely different ways. If you're at high risk, there's a strong rationale for taking both. If you're at moderate risk, a statin might be a much better bet. There's even a move afoot to make these cholesterol-lowering drugs available over the counter, as they are in England. "A statin a day" may well become the new motto for prevention in moderate-risk populations.

ANATOMY OF A HEART ATTACK

There are three key events: the formation of the blockage, then the fracturing of the blockage, and finally the formation of a blood clot.

Your coronary arteries are lined with flat, thin cells called endothelial cells. Imagine in your mind an old-style subway station, round in shape, lined with shiny ceramic tiles. Just as the tiles line the subway tunnel, these endothelial cells line the walls of your coronary arteries. Part of the endothelial cells' job is to prevent blood from leaking into the walls of the arteries while allowing nutrients to enter. Unfortunately, not only healthful nutrients can enter through these cells; bad cholesterol, technically termed LDL cholesterol, enters too. This LDL cholesterol slips through the endothelial cells and into a layer below it called the subendothelial layer. Imagine a leak under the tiles weakening the materials the tiles were meant to protect. Eventually the tiles bulge inward, break loose, and begin to collapse. This is essentially what happens with the buildup of LDL cholesterol under the endothelial cells.

If there is one villain to identify it is LDL cholesterol, an extremely toxic substance at the core of most heart attacks. Now let's look at the specifics.

After the LDL cholesterol seeps through into the area underlying the endothelial cells, it is attacked by a substance called a free radical. This causes the chemical reaction oxidation, which may be the most dangerous chemical reaction in your body. First, oxidation triggers the release of a variety of very small, intracellular chemicals termed cytokines. These cytokines are like poison daggers. They begin the process of creating blockages—called atherosclerotic plaques—in your arteries. Second, oxidation makes the LDL look like a foreign substance in the body. How? Just as we may be recognized by a name tag, cells are recognized by receptors on their surfaces. Once the immune system can no longer recognize LDL because it lacks that name tag or receptor, the immune system attacks the LDL. The attack is conducted by white blood cells called macrophages, acting just as they do when they attack a foreign body such as a splinter or a bacterium. If you remember the video game Pac-Man, these macrophages look like the little Pac-Men, gobbling up the LDL until they become engorged and eventually self-destruct. The cholesterol from them forms a large pool in the center of the plaque. This soft, squishy center grows larger and larger. This hot core of highly toxic LDL cholesterol is the heart of the problem.

The final blow occurs when a substance called metalloproteinase breaks down the material in the cap covering the plaque and causes it to thin and become vulnerable to fracture. The larger the soft spot in the middle, the more the plaque may be pushed around by the pressure of blood flowing by it. It is the fracture of this vulnerable plaque that is the catastrophic event that starts most heart attacks. When this happens, your chance of dying is one in four.

The new understanding of a heart attack is that the more unstable and prone to fracture the plaque is, the higher your risk. In fact, even small and seemingly innocuous plaques can fracture. Size is not the critical element.

This is the single most alarming new realization about heart attacks, especially for young and otherwise healthy people. With a small blockage, symptoms will be absent and a stress test will be negative. The greatest risk of heart attack comes from the rupture of small plaques. According to Dr. Paul Ridker, larger "mature" plaques are more stable and may in fact be *less* likely to rupture than smaller, presumably younger "less mature" plaques. Also, small plaques are much more common than large plaques.

This new explanation of heart attack lends itself to several forms of intervention. The most intriguing and alluring is a class of drugs called statins, which may reshape and stabilize the plaque to prevent it from fracturing. What makes the plaque unstable? A bigger cholesterol core. Statins can help to shrink that core. Unstable plaques also have thin caps that are more prone to fracture than thick and tough caps. This unstable plaque contains many inflammatory cells. Statins help both to drain the core and promote a thicker, more stable cap, while decreasing inflammation.

For decades we were concerned with slowing the growth of the plaque. Now there's a big new idea: stop it from fracturing. In most other areas of medicine, you'd have researchers going back to the lab to find the new miracle drug. Through great good fortune, it turns out that the very drugs most heart patients should be taking, statins, have a dramatic effect on this process. Statins decrease the risk of death from heart disease by a third or more. But here's where it gets interesting. The risk of death decreases very quickly after drug therapy is initiated. In fact, in some studies, the death rate decreases well before there is a substantial and long-lived decrease in cholesterol. That's what got researchers and clinicians thinking that statins just had to have an effect on the plaque's cap. Another class of drugs, called ACE inhibitors, also decreases the risk of death in heart attack patients. Again researchers believe that they stabilize the plaque.

This is the most complete picture to date of the classic heart attack. I think it's spectacular, since this new understanding gives us so many more effective ways of beating heart disease and doing it quickly—really quickly. As you'll see, statins and aspirin therapy reduce your risk in weeks, not years.

High levels of classic risk factors, however, may explain only about half of heart attack deaths. What explains the other half? Two key paths to heart attack are inflammation and a highly accelerated form of heart disease in a condition called metabolic syndrome. Yet in both of these conditions, your "bad" or LDL cholesterol can be near normal and you could easily escape detection. They account for a massive number of deaths each year and may explain a good chunk of the missing half.

INFLAMMATION

Fatal Flaw

Jack, a forty-nine-year-old investment banker, led the pack. He went to an Ivy League college and a top eastern business school. He belonged to all the best clubs. He was wealthy, had all the finest handmade English suits, and owned two vacation houses plus a late-model English luxury convertible. What he didn't have was a simple $20 blood test—a test that could have saved his life. He died suddenly and without warning from a massive heart attack.

His doctor, like many, had focused myopically on his cholesterol, which was normal. What killed him? Inflammation. As many as 35 million Americans are just like Jack. They have normal or moderately elevated cholesterol levels and are apparently healthy. However, also like Jack, they have sky-high levels of inflammation in their heart's arteries, putting them at unusually high risk of heart attack and stroke.

Conventional wisdom: My cholesterol is normal.
The real deal: Your CRP is out of the park.

We knew something was missing, and this is it, say the experts. "It" is inflammation. Doctors have long known that only about half of all heart attacks can be explained by traditional risk factors such as high cholesterol, high blood pressure, smoking, obesity, or lack of exercise. About half of the 1.1 million people who have heart attacks each year don't have high LDL cholesterol. A surprising and tragic number of people die never knowing that they had heart disease. Yet many do have inflammation, and lots of it, in their coronary arteries. Can this inflammation be measured just like cholesterol? Yes. There is a new test, which may soon be as familiar to you as that for cholesterol. It's called high sensitivity C-reactive protein or hsCRP. CRP is a key measure of the inflammation in your coronary arteries. Dr. Paul Ridker estimates that 25 percent of Americans have elevated levels of hsCRP even though they have normal or even low levels of cholesterol.

As the best measure of inflammation so far, hsCRP has proved to be a stronger predictor of cardiovascular disease than cholesterol in the largest study to date. It's a simple blood test for arterial inflammation shown to predict the risk of heart attack and stroke even in those with low cholesterol levels. Until recently, the hsCRP test was available only in specialty research centers and required special equipment to measure. However, just two years ago the test became widely available and can now be ordered by any physician during a routine cholesterol screening.

Why is inflammation important? You saw how a fractured plaque is the key event triggering a heart attack. By middle age, most of us have a fatty buildup of plaque in our coronary arteries, but what is it that makes that plaque more likely to fracture in some of us? Inflammation weakens plaque, making it far more fragile and prone to fracture.

On a more technical level, specialized white blood cells called macrophages fight infection. Macrophages gather inside plaques and begin to produce small chemicals and enzymes called metalloproteinases. These metalloproteinases break down the material in the cap, or surface, of the atherosclerotic plaque in the artery wall and cause it to fracture and break. One key chemical involved in the breakdown is CRP. Now that doctors can measure levels of CRP, they can measure the amount of inflammation taking place inside your plaques. When the plaque ruptures, all the clotting factors in the blood instantly react to the tissue factors below the surface of the vessel wall, and a large blood clot results. If that clot stubbornly clings to the surface of the artery wall, it will grow and block the entire vessel. That means that the heart muscle downstream of the blocked artery is suddenly and totally without blood, causing cell death in the heart muscle and what we call a heart attack.

As you saw earlier, the popular view of heart attacks was that arteries become narrower and narrower until they either are closed off completely or are blocked by a blood clot. Now comes the rather terrifying idea that you don't have to have much blockage at all. The plaque doesn't have to protrude deeply into your arteries to cause a heart attack. You simply have to have vulnerable plaques. Recent studies show that many people suffering heart attacks do *not* have severe blockages of their arteries. They have vulnerable plaques. When these vulnerable plaques break, they also promote the formation of blood clots, which block the arteries.

Inflammation, researchers believe, is the main reason that disease in the coronary arteries progresses and the vulnerability develops. This has led to a dramatic breakthrough in thinking about coronary artery disease. Rather than controlling the size of the plaque, the new goal is to stabilize the plaque so that its smaller size, smoother shape, and greater firmness protect against rupture. Draining the plaque of its cholesterol core also increases the stability of the plaque. Just as important, inflammation is reduced so that plaques don't become vulnerable.

Dr. Richard Stein, associate chair of the Department of Medicine at Beth Israel Medical Center, Herbert and Nell Singer Division, explains that most fractures actually occur on the outer perimeter of the plaque where plaque merges with noninvolved arterial wall—this is called the "shoulder" of the plaque. Three findings seem to play a role in a plaque becoming vulnerable.

1. Cells filled with cholesterol are found in large number at the shoulder area of the plaque.
2. The cap of the plaque thins out due to inflammation.
3. The cap over the plaque may become very vulnerable to fracture when increasing blood flow over and around it places great stress on it. The large cholesterol core is rela-

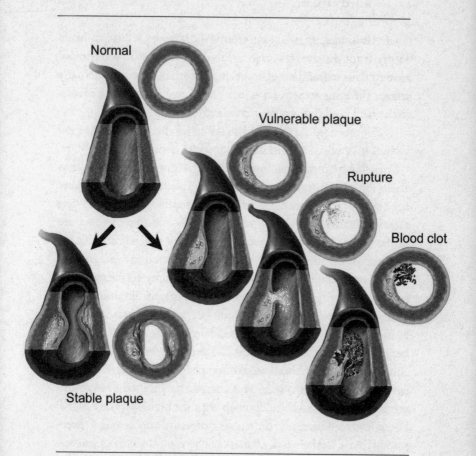

tively soft, giving rise to the term "soft spot." It is one of three pathologic traits found when examining a fractured plaque.

CRP is a significantly powerful risk factor. CRP is not just a signpost for disease. It is also involved in progression of the disease and in a number of molecular mechanisms that actually trigger the disease. So it's not just a marker; it's actually a mediator as well, and that makes it a target for treatment.

A pioneer in the field of hsCRP is Dr. Paul Ridker. He describes his biggest and most convincing scientific study to date. "We began by measuring hsCRP and along with cholesterol levels in 27,909 initially healthy women and then followed them for eight years to see who would eventually suffer from heart attacks and stroke. The bottom line is 77 percent of all future heart attacks and strokes occurred among women with an LDL cholesterol below 160 and 46 percent occurred in women with an LDL cholesterol below 130, the cut points physicians currently use as targets for prevention. This means that our federal guidelines are missing a huge number of individuals who are at high risk but are simply missed because we have not moved beyond cholesterol. Our study showed that hsCRP alone was actually a better marker of risk for heart attacks, strokes, and cardiovascular deaths than was the bad or LDL cholesterol. In our studies, both men and women with the highest levels of CRP had a fourfold increase in their risk of heart attack and a threefold increase in their risk of stroke. These risks were completely independent of other traditional risk factors such as high blood pressure, high cholesterol, smoking, or being overweight.

"Adding the hsCRP test to standard cholesterol screening must be where we go in the future," says Dr. Ridker. "The bottom line is that at any level of bad cholesterol, a high CPR is added risk. He adds that doctors "need to consider inflammation as a core way to think about risk and thus to better motivate our patients to take care of themselves." If doctors rely only on cholesterol to identify high-risk patients, they'll miss half of all patients with heart disease.

The biggest piece of missing evidence is proof that lowering CRP levels decreases the risk of heart disease. This was the same gap in the early days of lowering cholesterol. Everyone knew that lower cholesterol was better, but they had to prove that lowering it decreased the risk of heart attack and death. Even today, Dr. Claude Lenfant says that only statins have been proved to lower the risk of heart attack and death. To test this very issue, Dr. Ridker's group has just started a study of 15,000 middle-aged men and women to see if lowering CRP works as well as the experts believe it will. Patients who already have heart disease are also far more likely to run into trouble, like Vice President Dick Cheney. A recent study showed that patients with unstable chest pain due to coronary artery disease are at far higher risk if they have a high CRP. They're also more likely to develop calcium in their coronary arteries, a sure sign that cholesterol-laden blockages have grown and matured.

Based on the famous Framingham Heart Study, researchers found that "people with elevated CRP seemed to have or develop more coronary calcium, even after adjusting for age, traditional risk factors, and Framingham risk score." CRP measures inflammation, which is the process by which the body repairs itself. Calcium in the coronary arteries is an indicator of disease. Matching the two tests, as the Framingham researchers did, gives a rough correlation between inflammation levels and amount of coronary artery disease.

THE SOURCE OF INFLAMMATION

About half of those with a high CRP have a genetic predisposition to this inflammatory response. In the other half, inflammation may be related to poor diet, obesity, smoking, and lack of exercise. Dr. Paul Ridker hypothesizes that inflammation and heart disease go together just like inflammation and arthritis do. It becomes part and parcel of the disease.

HOW TO MEASURE INFLAMMATION

CRP is in your blood, so it can be measured with a very simple, inexpensive (about $20) blood test. The hsCRP test is now widely available in almost all patient care settings, including outpatient doctors' offices. Ask for it. hsCRP also turns out to be a very strong predictor not just of heart attacks and stroke but also of sudden cardiac death, peripheral arterial disease, and type 2 diabetes. Sudden cardiac death may be due to a massive heart attack or to sudden electrical instability.

Most experts say that you should have your CRP measured at the same time as your cholesterol. The reason hsCRP is exploding in clinical practice is that researchers have done very carefully designed studies demonstrating that an abnormal level when you're healthy predicts future risk of having a heart attack or other cardiovascular illness even if your cholesterol levels are low. Women with the highest CRP are six times more likely to have a heart attack than women with the lowest levels. Still, Dr. James Cleeman, director of the National Cholesterol Education Program, a federal program that aims to reduce coronary artery disease, has said, "Right now, they only have research implications." However, cardiologists who find high levels of hsCRP are sure to treat their patients far more aggressively. The test is particularly useful for those patients who don't have any warning flags for heart disease.

The bottom line is that a high hsCRP should motivate you and your physician to be much more aggressive in your care. hsCRP can show if you are at risk years before you would otherwise have your first heart attack. If you have moderate risk factors such as borderline high blood pressure or borderline cholesterol levels, or are simply middle-aged, there's even more reason to have the test. CRP's advocates say that everyone over forty should consider getting the test. In January 2003, the American Heart Association and United States Centers for Disease Control and Prevention issued recommendations for hsCRP testing in patients considered at moderate cardiovascular risk or when a physician is undecided about a course of treatment for a patient.

Vice President Dick Cheney had high hsCRP, but unfortunately he found this out only after he had suffered a series of life-threatening heart events. If he had known earlier, perhaps he would have been more aggressive in his care and his lifestyle: losing weight, increasing exercise, and modifying his diet. President Bush has his CRP measured regularly. His is quite low, consistent with his overall healthy profile and his regular exercise program.

High blood pressure and elevated levels of hsCRP may work together to increase cardiovascular risk in women, according to a study published in *Circulation*. Researchers found that when levels of both were elevated, the risk of heart attack and stroke increased as much as eight times. "This study provides the first evidence that hsCRP and blood pressure interact to increase the risk of adverse cardiovascular outcomes," said senior writer Paul Ridker.

The new findings strengthen the evidence that inflammation plays a key role in the development of cardiovascular disease. More important, baseline levels of CRP predict the future development of high blood pressure. There is the intriguing notion that inflammation is at the root of many diseases and that CRP may tip you off well before the development of not just high blood pressure and heart disease but also diabetes and stroke.

YOUR CRP TEST SCORE

The results of two tests, optimally two weeks apart, are averaged to provide a more stable estimate of CRP. If a level of > 10 mg/L is identified, your doctor should look for an obvious source of infection or inflammation; a cold and the flu can influence the result. A result of > 10 mg/L without such an obvious alternative cause is associated with a very high risk of heart disease.

An hsCRP value greater than 3 is considered high risk. Here are the cut points:

- Low risk: < 1 mg/L
- Average risk: 1 to 3 mg/L
- High risk: > 3 mg/L

Values above 3 mg/L carry about a threefold increase in relative risk compared with the low-risk group. Individuals with LDL cholesterol below 130 mg/dL who have CRP levels above 3 mg/L represent a high-risk group often missed in clinical practice. "In fact," Dr. Ridker states, "such individuals may represent the great majority of the nearly half million heart attacks and strokes that occur each year among those with normal cholesterol levels." My LDL is very low, but my CRP is high normal. This has certainly motivated me!

TREATMENT

The idea of inflammation as a cause of heart disease is new, but there are potential treatments. By far the most important are lifestyle changes. Exercise, weight loss, smoking cessation are all known to lower cardiac risk, and they all also lower hsCRP levels. In addition, drugs can help.

There are no large, long-term studies yet, but, says Dr. Jeffrey Borer, "the data are very suggestive." What do you do about inflammation? Here's a look.

ANTI-INFLAMMATORY DRUGS

These cut inflammation throughout your body, from sore knees to sprained ankles. They work the same way in your heart's arteries.

Aspirin is used daily by many heart patients. If you are already taking aspirin, you are deriving a secondary benefit—decreased inflammation in your heart's arteries. Aspirin works better to prevent heart attacks in people with higher CRPs than lower CRPs, as demonstrated in a 1997 randomized, double-blind, placebo-controlled trial conducted by Dr. Ridker.

The usual recommended dose is one baby aspirin (81 mg) a day. The optimum dose of aspirin for decreasing inflammation is not known. Primary and secondary prevention trials have demonstrated benefits with a variety of regimes including 75 mg per day, 100 mg per day, and 325 mg every other day. Doses of 75 mg per day appear as effective as higher doses, and have a lower risk of the main complication of aspirin, bleeding from the stomach.

Statins are the powerful drugs that lower your cholesterol level. They also reduce inflammation. From a very practical vantage point, that means that many people on the fence about taking statins now ought to consider them. Paul Ridker reiterates, "Statins do two things of interest: They both lower CRP levels, and they again appear to be more effective in terms of preventing heart attacks when the CRP levels are high. That means that the statins are kind of like twofers—they lower LDL *and* they lower CRP levels. This is extremely interesting." Statins work both for those who have never had a heart attack and those who have. Dr. Ridker has embarked on an extraordinary experiment: using cholesterol-lowering drugs to treat patients who have low cholesterol but have high CRP.

Dr. Ridker says that statins are the most important drugs to treat high CRP. Studies with pravastatin, lovastatin, simvastatin, and atorvastatin have all shown that, on average, median CRP levels decline 15 to 25 percent as soon as six weeks after initiation of therapy.

EXPERT ADVICE
Dr. Richard Stein: "Statins are the only effective drug that lowers CRP. As the CRP got higher, the risk got higher. Statins would bring those values down by almost 20 to 30 percent."

COX-2 inhibitors have had their share of controversy. Originally touted to lower the risk of stomach bleeding, later studies have cast some doubt on how much that risk is decreased. There has also been a risk of heart attack alleged in past studies. However, a preliminary Swiss study from University Hospital in Zurich shows that COX-2 inhibitors such as Celebrex reduce CRP levels, reduce inflammation, and improve the function of blood vessels.

Other medications such as ACE inhibitors and the antiplatelet drug clopidogrel (Plavix), may also decrease inflammation. Newly released data show that TZDs (new drugs that help glucose cross into cells, thereby lowering blood sugar levels) also reduce inflammation "dramatically," says Dr. Steven Nissen. He adds that there is research being done on other anti-inflammatory drugs, but nothing is known at this point and they are not currently recommended for cardiac inflammation.

Dr. Dennis L. Sprecher, formerly of the Cleveland Clinic Foundation and currently the director of dyslipidemia at Discovery Medicine's Cardiovascular and Urogenital Department, adds this fascinating note: "So maybe we believe that inflammation is part of our overall aging process and therefore many people should go on an anti-inflammatory cocktail as soon as they reach age fifty or before. This may lead to some benefit with regards to dementia and other functional abnormalities and maybe even cancers, since we really don't understand the etiologies of many of these commons disorders that end up in our demise."

HEALTHY LIVING

Diet and weight loss, exercise, and smoking cessation are the most important things you can do to reduce hsCRP levels. Dr. Paul Ridker adds that moderate alcohol consumption can also decrease CRP, as can control of high blood pressure. Using CRP as a barometer of your heart health is a new and novel motivator and scoring system to keep track of your progress. Even weight loss by itself is a great way to lower CRP.

INFLAMMATION AND HEART FAILURE

Inflammation may damage the heart muscle directly, leading to heart failure. The Canadian pharmaceutical company Vasogen has begun a trial to test its anti-inflammatory drug Celacade, to determine if it reduces death and hospitalizations for patients with heart failure.

Inflammation is easy to beat. Be sure to have your CRP level measured and then act on it; then have it retested in six to eight weeks to check your progress. Everything you need to know about damping the inflammation in your coronary arteries is contained in Step 6, "Take Lifesaving Medications." Throughout this book, I look at those patients who fall through the cracks, who suffer heart attacks and die before their heart disease is detected. Inflammation and high hsCRP levels are certain to explain tens of thousands of heart attacks in patients who otherwise are at low risk. CRP is cheap. There's no harm in knowing your CRP level and potentially great benefit to be derived from lowering it.

ACCELERATOR

Fatal Flaw

A hardy New Englander, Fred lived a robust and good life. He was fun, athletic, and successful. I'd known him since college. He knew enough about heart disease to have his cholesterol checked, which was normal, even a little low. That's why the chest discomfort one winter's afternoon caused little concern. The pain intensified, alarming his wife and children. "It's nothing," he said. Nevertheless, his concerned family brought him to a hospital, where the EKG showed a massive and lethal heart attack. Despite the best efforts of a major medical center, he died that afternoon.

The Monday morning quarterbacks pored over his medical records. It was all there. He'd gained a little weight over the last stressful year, after he began a new job, accounting for his increased abdominal girth. Sure, his cholesterol was great, but another blood fat, called a triyglyderide, was out of the ballpark. His blood sugar had attracted little attention during his annual physical—it was high but hardly alarming. His blood pressure too was mildly elevated. And his good cholesterol, just drawn the previous week, was low. Put the pieces together and the diagnosis, with twenty-twenty hindsight, was obvious. Once called syndrome X because of its mysterious qualities, it's now called metabolic syndrome. To the embarrassment of his physician, his case was classic and easily treatable in such a motivated and health-conscious patient.

They call metabolic syndrome the elephant because it's known only by its tusks, or trunk, or tail. Most doctors don't see the whole syndrome, just pieces of it, until it's too late. They're far more likely to miss it than not, and that's a potential tragedy. It multiplies your risk factors, each of which may appear small or even insignificant on its own. I call it the accelerator because it can lay down a plaque with a speed that is frightening even in young, previously healthy men and women—months, not years. According to the American Heart Association's statistics, in 2004 a stunning 49 million Americans have metabolic syndrome, making it the most frequent and least known of all major illnesses. By age sixty, as many as 60 percent of Americans will have metabolic syndrome.

Conventional wisdom: My blood tests are pretty good, not perfect, but good enough.
The real deal: Multiple small abnormalities can add up and kill you.

The poisonous mixture inside Fred's coronary arteries was radically altered by metabolic syndrome, which rapidly accelerated the growth of blockages in the worst possible place—the origin of the left anterior descending coronary artery. The risk translated into a lethal blockage in one of his main coronary arteries. In other patients, these blockages can grow from undetectable to lethal in months.

Fred's arteries were in pretty good shape in every place but the most important place. In very fast-moving, turbulent sections of coronary arteries, blockages can build up fast, and that's precisely where his fatal blockage was. The harsh eddies and undercurrents found at the fork of a fast-moving river can quickly build up sandbars and silt deposits. That's what happened in Fred.

What's the lesson drawn from this? Look at the whole picture. Treat small abnormalities early and aggressively.

METABOLIC SYNDROME

The truth is that doctors don't know exactly what metabolic syndrome is. They know how to define it, like a blind person feeling the tusks, legs, and ears of an elephant. But like the blind man, they can't see it. So the disease is still in the process of being defined. What they do know is that it is highly dangerous and that it can be measured. Patients run into trouble because their doctors, like the blind man, find too few parts to see the big picture. Medical charts often contain all the information necessary to make the diagnosis, but the health care provider frequently fails to put all the data together to form the big picture. More commonly, too few measurements are taken so that the basic information is not there to make the diagnosis. With just a few simple tests, you can easily determine if you fit into metabolic syndrome.

Here's what to look for:

- Overweight with fat distribution in the abdominal region
- Elevated fasting triglycerides

- Low HDL cholesterol
- High blood pressure
- Elevated fasting blood glucose

If just one or two of these factors are elevated, that's not enough. The World Health Organization and the National Cholesterol Education Program require three of the five features to make the diagnosis of metabolic syndrome. There is, however, one risk factor they all have in common. Everyone with metabolic syndrome is technically obese: just a 40-inch waist in men, 35 inches in women.

Note that LDL cholesterol is not included, and that's what makes it so incredibly easy to miss metabolic syndrome. If you have only your total cholesterol measured, your doctor will miss it. He or she won't detect either the high triglyceride or the low HDL measurement. Commonly, your health care provider will see a small increase in blood pressure and a little elevation in blood sugar, and say things look just fine or at best tell you to watch your diet.

All five hallmarks of the metabolic syndrome are independently and significantly linked to heart attack and stroke, according to the NHANES III national survey. Let's look at each of them in depth.

ABDOMINAL FAT

If you store a good deal of your fat around your midsection, you have what is called an apple body type, as opposed to the pear shape found in people who store more fat in their buttocks and thighs. Fat around the tummy is called metabolically active, meaning that it has a major effect on the fats in your blood that could lead to a heart attack.

Measure your waist with a tape measure around the area above your hip bone and below your rib cage. You have abdominal obesity if you are a man and your waist is more than 40 inches, or if you are a woman with a waist of more than 35 inches. If your waist measurement exceeds these numbers, and your BMI (body mass index) is above 25, you have an increased risk of developing type 2 diabetes, hypertension, and cardiovascular disease, according to the American Obesity Association.

It's easy to determine your BMI. Divide your weight in pounds by your height in inches squared. Multiply that number by 703. Here's an example of a man 5'10" (70") who weighs 200 pounds. $200 \div 4,900 = 0.0408 \times 703 =$ a BMI of 28.7. Or check the chart in the Appendix, page 261.

TRIGLYCERIDES

Triglycerides are an often overlooked and misunderstood component of any comprehensive test of your blood fats. If you have only your cholesterol measured, you could miss a big part of the picture. Triglycerides are the most common type of fat in the body. Your body uses triglycerides for energy and stores them as body fat for future use. If, after an overnight fast, your blood triglyceride level is over 150, you fall farther into metabolic syndrome.

Non-HDL testing is becoming a popular way to target people with metabolic syndrome because it detects unusually high triglyceride levels. Ask your doctor if he or she can test for it.

LOW HDL

HDL is the "good" cholesterol that reflects the ability of your blood to remove dangerous levels of fats and protect your arteries from the buildup of plaques. If your HDL is too low, you lack a significant ability to protect yourself against heart attack. Low HDL is below 40 in men or below 50 in women. HDL should be part of your cholesterol screening. With an HDL of 20, heart disease is almost unavoidable.

HIGH BLOOD PRESSURE

Normal blood pressure is considered to be 110/70. Any level over 130/85 is enough to put you squarely into metabolic syndrome.

HIGH FASTING BLOOD GLUCOSE

This is the clincher. If, after an overnight fast, your blood sugar level is over 110, you have the final diagnostic criterion for metabolic syndrome. On its own, blood sugar of 110 is not very alarming. People with badly out of control diabetes can have blood sugar up to 800. So if you settle out at 115, it's not much of an attention getter. I've viewed thousands of reports marked up by doctors with comments like "good going" and "keep up the good work" because the values of the above tests are so close to normal. Don't be fooled. If any of your readings is outside of the correct range, you should keep an eye out for metabolic syndrome. The high blood sugar is the driving force behind metabolic syndrome since it causes both low HDL and high triglycerides.

Dr. Paul Ridker notes that within the next year CRP is likely to be added to the definition of metabolic syndrome. If you have the above risks, the higher your CRP, the higher your overall risk. This firmly connects CRP to metabolic syndrome and demonstrates that inflammation is part and parcel of it.

Let's sum this up with a simple checklist.

Defining Risk Factor	Criterion for Metabolic Syndrome
Abdominal obesity	> 40" waist in men
	> 35" waist in women
High fasting triglycerides	≥ 150 mg/dL
Low HDL	< 40 mg/dL for men
	< 50 mg/dL for women
High blood pressure	≥ 130/85 mmHg
High fasting blood glucose	> 110 mg/dL

THE TOTAL PACKAGE

If all three of your values in the checklist are above normal, including abdominal obesity, you have metabolic syndrome. Each risk may seem minor on its own. However, if you have the whole package, you have a lot to worry about. Patients gain a false sense of comfort from health care providers who do not appreciate the significance of these multiple seemingly minor findings. Who doesn't have a little bit too big a ring around the middle? Whose blood pressure isn't up a notch? Whose good cholesterol doesn't stray below normal? Not bad, you might say.

You ignore metabolic syndrome at your peril. You can see how doctors can be misled or easily miss metabolic syndrome. The result, however, of missing metabolic syndrome often ends in tragedy. Remember that the first symptom of heart attack is often sudden death. Metabolic syndrome accounts for a major number of those sudden deaths, what I call in this book the missing half. This high-risk group has not been tapped for diagnosis or treatment. Says Dr. Luther Clark, chief of cardiology at the State University of New York, Downstate Medical Center, "There are many people out there who figure, well, a little high blood pressure, a little high cholesterol, and a little overweight. I only have to worry about this a little. In fact, they need to worry a lot. These people either have a false sense of comfort themselves, or the physicians who take care of them may not appreciate the significance of all these multiple minor things." Discover if you have metabolic syndrome and you could save your life.

This is a silent syndrome destined to kill millions of Americans. Still, metabolic syndrome accounts for only some of the patients with elevated blood sugar levels. The bigger and much more obvious epidemic is of adult-onset diabetes. Diabetes is a lethal accelerator of coronary artery disease, where new blockages can develop in months, not years. We're seeing the beginning of a major and explosive epidemic of diabetes. One-third of children born today will be diabetic if American lifestyles stay on their present course. Diabetes itself can often be easily detected by a simple fasting blood test. Experts no longer believe that it's okay if you have "just a little bit of sugar." If your blood sugar is elevated at all, it's simply a matter of the degree of diabetes you have.

Says Dr. Dennis Sprecher, "The very simple rule of thumb is that having metabolic syndrome is not necessarily equivalent to having diabetes, because a lot of people think that diabetes has a very specific cut point. But doctors are realizing that the clinical problems that we see in association with diabetes and metabolic syndrome represent a continuum, relegating the idea of a hard cut point to a practical but perhaps misleading clinical nuance."

With diabetes, symptoms of a heart attack are often abnormal or missing, which is why diabetics need to focus so intently on reducing their risks. Both diabetics and those with metabolic syndrome need to move to the most aggressive medical therapy possible because of the terrifying speed with which blockages can develop. The most alarming aspect of metabolic syndrome was revealed at a 2003 American Heart Association conference, where Dr. Joanne Harrell, director of the Center for Research on Chronic Illness at the University of North Carolina School of

Nursing, reported that one in eight schoolchildren already has three or more risk factors for metabolic syndrome. She fears that if nothing is done for these children, a good number will develop diabetes and heart disease.

In the hunt for the missing half in adults, metabolic syndrome already accounts for the most easily missed warning signs. I was shocked when my blood was tested and the results showed my triglycerides and blood sugar toward the high end of normal and my HDL low. Even the most heart conscious of us can veer toward metabolic syndrome, as I learned after a stressful year in Iraq. What is reassuring is that strict attention to diet and exercise can beat metabolic syndrome. I am being a lot more careful now!

Remember, metabolic syndrome is a lifestyle disease that can be treated *and even cured* simply with rigorous diet, exercise, and lifestyle changes.

STEP TWO: KNOW THE WARNING SIGNS

"I'm afraid he's not. We've worked on him for nearly an hour, but we can't get his heart started again. I just wanted to tell you that we've tried everything we can." I reassured her, "You did everything you could. Thank you for all your efforts on your husband's behalf."

She smiled faintly, then turned and walked away.

I'll never forget looking inside his wallet for prescriptions and medical alert data. He had been in some financial difficulty. There were multiple dunning notices in his wallet, now so irrelevant. His last days had been anything but pleasant. The warning signs had been there, but he, his wife, and his physician had missed them, perhaps distracted by financial troubles.

Many patients never get an early warning. Of the 1.5 million heart attacks each year, the latest Centers for Disease Control statistics show that between 400,000 and 460,000 result in sudden cardiac death. For many, the first symptom of coronary artery disease is the last—sudden death. In this chapter I look at the key symptoms and warning signs of a heart attack and sudden death you need to know about, many of which are quite surprising. When you finish this chapter, you'll have a better understanding of why so many of the missing half never come forward in time.

Conventional wisdom: Sharp, crushing chest pain means you're having a heart attack.
The real deal: Symptoms are often subtle, misleading, and even absent.

This well-trained nurse missed a heart attack in her own husband. Even in the case of my father, a Harvard Medical School graduate, the significance of his symptoms was overlooked. The evening he died, he had excessive fatigue and couldn't stay awake for his favorite show, *Wall Street Week,* at 8:30. We'll never know what other symptoms he suffered, since he kept them to himself. The fact is, he wasn't feeling well. He also had an eerie premonition that he was going to die. Instead of going to the hospital's emergency department, he went to bed. Knowing the symptoms and acting quickly is the biggest single lifesaving measure you can take to avoid dying from a heart attack.

Most of us expect a heart attack to scream out at us with the classical crushing chest pain beneath the sternum, radiating down the left arm and accompanied by a soaking sweat and nausea. If it were that easy, we'd all be cardiologists. A massive heart attack in a young person could present with those symptoms because there is a sudden and massive occlusion (blockage) of a single coronary artery.

But most of us aren't that lucky. "The classical symptoms are easy," says Dr. Steven Nissen. "A man in his fifties has gripping pain in the center of his chest, with the pain spreading up to his jaw and out to his left arm, accompanied by shortness of breath, nausea, and a cold sweat. Unless he's got an incredible power of denial, he knows he's got coronary disease and is suffering a major heart attack. The real problem is patients presenting in atypical ways. Tragically, the numbers of those patients are enormous."

What makes a great cardiologist is the ability to pick through those very nondescript, vague, and atypical symptoms. I don't want to turn you into a hypochondriac, but *any* new unexplained symptoms in the chest or upper abdomen should make you consider heart disease.

The most alarming data come out of the Cleveland Clinic in studies of potential heart transplant donors. An astonishing 85 percent of sixty-year-olds already had coronary artery disease, yet very few had any symptoms. To be perfectly clear, if you're a man over fifty or a woman over sixty, chances are very high that you already have heart disease even if you don't have symptoms. So how will you know?

KNOW THE SYMPTOMS

Since symptoms vary tremendously, I've asked top cardiologists to sort through the tricky kinds of symptoms that heart patients present with. Says Steven Nissen, "It's subtle. I will tell you that the average family practitioners aren't going to be able to do this. They just don't quite get it, and that's a really big problem." This chapter will alert you to the most subtle symptoms.

Dr. Jeffrey Borer often asks patients if they have any discomfort in their chest area. "What I get back is, 'I don't have any pain, Doc.' I didn't say pain, what I asked about was discomfort or abnormal sensation in the chest." Don't wait until it hurts to see your doctor. Physicians have to persist and take a detailed history to determine if someone has symptoms that might be associated with heart disease. And it's not only abnormal sensation in the chest, it's also difficulty breathing, light-headedness, palpitations, feeling faint. Even when severely ill, my mother only complained of vague light-headedness and shortness of breath. Those are the symptoms you need to share with your physician. Many busy primary care practitioners just don't have the time to ask or don't know to ask the right questions.

Jeffrey Borer says, "Just checking someone's cholesterol is real nice and done all the time, but that's not the first step. I go to health fairs all the time. I see lots of people lined up for blood pressure measurements or cholesterol tests. What's missed is that no one asks them if they have chest pain, trouble with exercise, shortness of breath. This may be the biggest single mistake in all of cardiology. So many patients believe that cholesterol is the whole game when in fact there can be lots else going on." Let's take a look at what top cardiologists have to sort through.

INDIGESTION

Indigestion is the most confusing complaint. The number of men and women who have gone to their graves believing they just "ate something that didn't agree with them" is legion—just like the man I described at the opening of this chapter. Even patients who normally have some reflux of the stomach's acid into the esophagus, called gastroesophageal reflux disease, often cannot distinguish heart pain from reflux disease. Many heart patients have both diseases and it's very hard for them to figure out which disease is causing the symptoms.

Here's why. Heart pain and esophageal pain are visceral, that is, they come from your internal organs. There's a major difference between visceral pain and somatic pain, what you feel on your skin. When you get a splinter in your finger, you know exactly where it is and you have a pretty good idea what it is, just from feel. That's because there is a specific pain fiber at that exact point on the skin, which takes the message to the brain. However, the pain fibers coming from internal organs are imprecise and don't tell the brain very accurately where the pain is coming from. Those fibers can give the same symptom whether the pain is coming from the heart, esophagus, stomach, or other internal organ. That creates a huge challenge for doctors. Dr. James Atkins of the University of Texas Southwestern Medical Center says, "That's why we miss heart attacks in the emergency department at times—because the symptoms sound more like reflux disease."

IMPENDING DOOM

Classic heart attack victims do not drop in horror, clutching their chests, as we see in movies. They often sit quietly with a frightening feeling of impending doom. This is exactly what my father suffered in the two days before he died. He wrote final letters to his children. Again, since his doctor had counseled him that he would never have a heart attack, and since he had never been warned of the symptoms, he failed to seek medical care. He's not alone. As many as 60 to 80 percent of people who have heart attacks have some premonitory symptoms. What's truly amazing is that those symptoms are perceived somewhere between forty-eight and seventy-two hours before the event—and in some cases four to six *weeks* before.

FATIGUE

If you find that you are becoming fatigued with progressively less exertion, you may well have a key early warning sign of heart disease. And if you find yourself too tired to do things you usually do easily, watch out. This is a key symptom of a heart attack.

Though there are many causes of fatigue, one of them is severe coronary artery disease not associated with chest discomfort or pain. Says Jeffrey Borer, "Abnormal fatigability would be a subtle symptom that would suggest the possibility of important cardiac disease long before some cataclysmic event occurs." Here's one chilling fact: In a study of people who had died suddenly, the most common symptom was fatigue. Harvard's Dr. Thomas Graboys confirms that: "The most common symptom that my patients talk to me about is their fatigue. Therefore, any exertional symptom, whether it's exertional throat discomfort or chest or arm that comes with exposure to the cold for example or when it's very humid and abates when you slow down the pace, the burden of responsibility now is on me to say that isn't coming from the heart."

Dr. Claude Lenfant emphasizes above all else the importance of fatigue as a symptom. If you are uncharacteristically tired and feel fatigued, realize that you may be on the brink of having a heart attack.

Fatigue is a key symptom in women. A recent study of women who had heart attacks showed that 95 percent experienced some warning signs a month before their attack.

Researchers question patients whose heart attacks were discovered long after the fact on routine examinations. Patients are prodded about symptoms they ignored. Fully half describe having nondescript symptoms, such as being fatigued for as long as six weeks before the heart attack. In other words, they were tipped off but failed to tell their doctor. If you report increasing fatigue, your doctor can order a specific test to determine if your heart is the origin of your symptoms and then take measures to prevent the heart attack from occurring.

CHEST SENSATIONS

Crushing chest pain is the warning sign most of us have seen on *ER,* but it's far more important to be aware of other abnormal chest sensations. Most of the cardiologists I spoke to agree that *any* abnormal sensation in the region of the chest is a potential indicator that something is going on." If you mention unusual sensations in the chest to your doctor, your chance of detecting a coronary event before some tragedy occurs is greatly increased. The sensation doesn't have to be in the middle of the front of the chest, where you put your fist on your chest and say, "I feel pressure here." That may be typical, but any symptom in or around the chest that occurs with exertion and goes away with rest is suspect. Take the case of one of Jeffrey Borer's patients.

He was "trotting" across the park and had discomfort across his upper back. He stopped and the discomfort went away, but when he started again, the discomfort across his upper back came back. He called a friend of his who's a doctor but not a cardiologist, who surmised that there was something wrong and referred him to Dr. Borer. "I heard this piece of a story and I had the man come in. I got a typical story of exertion-related back pain. We sent him to the catheterization lab later that day, where we found he had severe three-vessel coronary artery disease. He was operated on the next day."

I've seen patients who have pain only in the jaw or arm or neck or chest. If you have a new sensation on exertion, tell your doctor. Says Dr. Thomas Graboys, "When you get angina, it's really not pain. Angina is a pressure or burning or tightness, but it's not a pain. If you can point to it, that takes it away from it being related to the heart. It falls in the category of musculoskeletal. But frankly, when in doubt, it's much better to be conservative and admit the patient to the hospital and keep an eye on him for a night."

Dr. James Atkins says, "People look for the so-called Hollywood heart attack—John Wayne suddenly grasping his chest in extreme pain and collapsing to the floor. That's not the way it presents. A lot of times, it's slow and insidious, comes and goes, and the person has a lot of problems figuring out what it is." Steven Nissen agrees: "If I go down to the emergency department to see a patient and he's writhing in pain, it's probably not a heart attack. It's not writhing pain; it's not like an acute gallbladder attack. A heart attack patient is often lying very quietly; he has a look of fear and doom on his face. He's not really saying much. He has this look, and the pain is not really agonizing. That's one of the problems. It's boring, it's dull. It can be very severe, but it isn't the kind of stabbing, writhing pain you get from other disorders." Dr. Joseph Ornato emphasizes, "We try not to use the word 'pain.' That's a big thing to really home in on again because of the Hollywood heart attack image that people have of tightness or pressure or a squeezing-type of sensation. The image is wrong on two counts, both in the character of the discomfort—usually it is gradual onset of a dull ache—and the fact that heart attack patients don't collapse to the ground unless they develop a complication called cardiac arrest."

In fact, in the majority of "heart attacks," if victims have any symptoms at all, the most common one is chest discomfort. That's borne out by the Framingham study, which over forty years has found chest discomfort the most typical symptom. The problem is, most people ignore these symptoms and only in retrospect say, "Oh, yes, I had some discomfort in my chest but it wasn't really pain, Doc. It was just a funny feeling."

If you learn one key point in this chapter, it is that the symptoms of a heart attack, in most cases, are *not* classic. "Pain" is the word used on TV dramas, not in cardiologists' offices. Good cardiologists never ask people about pain; they ask about abnormal sensations. People define in their heads what pain associated with a heart attack should be. Since most of them have never had a heart attack, they have no idea what it's supposed to be, but they have a bias that it must be some sharp, excruciating pain. Again, pain is their perception; the actual concern to a doctor is, "Did you feel something different in your chest today than you felt yesterday?"

However, many patients have no chest symptoms at all. This phenomenon is especially common in women, 43 percent of whom have no chest discomfort. This may explain why heart attacks are missed more commonly in women than men.

LIGHT-HEADEDNESS

"You should be very concerned about the possibility of heart disease if you feel faint or light-headed, particularly during or after exertion," says Steven Nissen. "Gosh, if I had a dollar for every old person who came into the emergency department and said, 'You know, I was feeling okay and next thing I knew I was very dizzy and found myself on the floor.' Then I ask, 'Did you have chest pain?' 'No.' 'Did you have shortness of breath?' 'No.' I give them an electrocardiogram and see a big heart attack. Some older folks just get short of breath or they may feel extreme lethargy or tiredness."

SHORTNESS OF BREATH

Shortness of breath can be the main or only symptom.

NEW SYMPTOMS

If you already have heart disease, then the new onset of chest pain should be a cause for action. Something has changed in your coronary arteries.

ATYPICAL SYMPTOMS

Diabetics are more likely to have atypical symptoms because diabetes impairs the ability of nerves to sense pain. Diabetes can damage both sensory and autonomic nerves. The autonomic nerves sense the generalized discomfort from the heart muscle trying to travel up the pain pathways to the brain. Diabetes may scramble these signals, leading to atypical symptoms.

Older patients and, to some extent, women tend to present with less typical symptoms than middle-aged men. The older you are, the more likely you are to have atypical symptoms, but it is still true that even in the highest age ranges chest discomfort is the most common symptom.

"The problem with the kinds of symptoms one might think about is that they're so highly nonspecific," says Dr. Jeffrey Borer. "They could mean ten other things." Adds Dr. Thomas Graboys, "The biggest problem is misdiagnosis both at the patient and the physician level. This means that the patient is experiencing some symptoms that he or she interprets as 'indigestion' and comes in and there's no EKG change and the patient feels okay and is sent home. And then the person comes back in either cardiac arrest or with a heart attack." In Dr. Graboys's office, everyone encourages patients that if symptoms are at all ambiguous, it's better to let your physician take responsibility to determine if something is going on or not.

Here's the most incredible irony. A large fraction of patients saw their physician within a month prior to dying of a heart attack. They knew something was going on, but neither they nor their physician could sort through the vague symptoms they were having to determine that they had heart disease and were about to suffer a heart attack.

Cardiologists are always on the alert for patients who complain of just weakness, tiredness, sweating, shortness of breath, fainting, GI-type nausea, or vomiting. Dr. Joseph Ornato tells his paramedics, nurses, and other doctors that when they get a patient "who is older and doesn't look right, is a little pale, looks sick, is a little short of breath, and sweaty, maybe a little sick to the stomach," to do an echocardiogram immediately, even if there isn't tightness or pressure in the chest. He adds, "About one-quarter of heart attack victims have atypical symptoms—face or jaw pain, fatigue, or nausea."

Women commonly have atypical symptoms such as upper abdominal pain, lower chest pain, and nausea. The diagnosis of heart attack is commonly missed. One of my best friends from my childhood felt extremely ill. She went to the hospital in the afternoon, believing she was suffering a heart attack. After an evaluation, she was sent home. The next morning she was found dead in the shower.

SILENT HEART ATTACK

Heart disease is often a silent killer, like an assassin. That's why risk factor assessment and stress testing become so important. Just as colon cancer can often be silent, so can heart disease. There's even a name for it: subclinical heart disease. The statistic is astounding: About a quarter of heart attacks are silent. That is, they are not associated with the typical abnormal chest sensations. They're discovered only later when someone looks at an electrocardiogram and sees evidence of an old heart attack, or after the sudden death of the patient. Half of patients with silent heart attacks recalled no symptoms at all in the previous two years. And women are at highest risk of having an undetected first heart attack, according to a famous study in the *New England Journal of Medicine:* "When heart attack was the first coronary event, nearly half were unrecognized in women, compared to only one-third undetected in men. Both men and women with unrecognized heart attacks usually presented with no symptoms at the time of the attack or had symptoms so atypical that neither they nor their physician suspected a heart attack."

Your best hope of avoiding a silent heart attack is a very thorough evaluation of your risk factors and further testing to uncover disease if your risk factors trigger suspicion. Dr. Claude Lenfant emphasizes that above all else, make sure your doctor is talking to you and asking you if you have chest pain, trouble with exercise, shortness of breath, unusual fatigue.

Who is most likely to have a silent heart attack? Diabetics, who have an altered ability to sense pain coming from the heart and those with left ventricular hypertrophy. (In LVH, the muscle of the main pumping chamber of the heart is thickened; it may or may not be enlarged. This is detected by physical exam, EKG, and echocardiogram. See Step 5, "Get the Right Diagnosis".)

DENIAL

The one finding most victims of heart disease share is denial. Take a middle-aged man who has a history of high blood pressure and high cholesterol, and is experiencing exertional chest discomfort. By definition, he most probably has coronary disease and is receiving a telegram. But the question is whether or not he is paying attention to the telegram. Dr. Thomas Graboys says that people usually notice that something is going on. The problem is that too many of them don't pick up the phone and talk to their doctor and figure out what to do.

Are you a denier? Take this brief quiz from the American Heart Association. The more yes answers, the bigger denier you are.

- I'll be embarrassed if it's just heartburn.
- I'm not sure if my pain fits the warning signs.
- I'm too young to have a heart attack.
- The pain's not that bad. I'll wait a while and see if it goes away.
- Only men get heart attacks.
- I'm as healthy as a horse.
- I can't be having a heart attack.

Clinical psychologists who study this phenomenon say it isn't so much just "denial," it's really "loss of control."

MISSED DIAGNOSIS

Despite all the advances in emergency care, up to 80,000 patients a year get sent home from the emergency department with an undiagnosed heart attack. If you are being dismissed from an emergency department with any of the symptoms listed on pages 57–58, insist on further observation or more definitive testing before going home.

We doctors make mistakes, and we listen carefully to concerned patients. Patients who get sent home with a heart attack have a reasonably high risk; 20 to 30 percent of them will die in the next six weeks. Missed heart attacks account for about 20 percent of malpractice dollars paid by emergency physicians. That's the largest single category—more than missed fractures or mistreated trauma. Missed heart attacks are on the rise in doctors' offices, especially primary care providers rather than cardiologists. There's a matching shift in lawsuits lodged against primary care physicians who have missed a heart attack. Experts insist that it's not because primary care physicians are bad doctors. Rather, so many more primary care physicians are seeing so many more patients. Over the last five to ten years, the increase in HMOs and primary care physicians has led many more patients to seek help first from their primary care physician or local health clinic rather than the emergency room. Heart attacks are also missed because emergency room crews let their guard down.

Only about 15 percent of patients coming to an emergency room with chest pain are actually having a heart attack. Furthermore, as few as 4 percent of chest pain patients are truly urgent cases who need to be rushed into the cath lab or given clot busters. This causes negative reinforcement in the hospital staff. Chest pain patients take a lot of work for doctors and nurses to evaluate as quickly as possible.

Since most people in the ER aren't having a heart attack, over time, the staff lets its guard down. Doctors are far less likely to drop everything and run when another person with chest pain comes into the ER than when a gunshot victim comes in. That's why you need to be a vigilant health care consumer. Be aware of your symptoms. Express your reservations. Be sure all the correct tests are done. You may also be at risk because of your age. Says Dr. Bruce MacLeod, chairman of the Department of Emergency Medicine at Mercy Hospital in Pittsburgh, "The reasons heart attacks are missed are usually that the patients are at the extremes of age. I've seen a woman at twenty-five have a myocardial infarction. She had bad genes, which contributed, but that case shows that it can happen. I took care of a patient who was thirty and a runner who came in with an MI. If for some reason you're not attuned to the possibility of an MI at a young age, you can miss someone who's young and having symptoms of a heart attack. Or the other extreme of age. A ninety-year-old man, for example, comes in with just weakness, and we don't immediately think heart attack. It's the extremes of age that seem to be where myocardial infarctions are missed now."

I've described a large range of presentations and symptoms for a heart attack. I sum them up in the following lists of symptoms. Which are you most likely to have? Dr. James Atkins says that the rule of thirds applies to those who are admitted to the hospital. About one-third have chest pain as the main symptom. Another third have shortness of breath, weakness, dizziness, or passing out as the main symptom along with chest pain. One-third of those who come to the hospital with a heart attack don't have chest pain at all.

TYPICAL SYMPTOMS
- Any abnormal sensation such as pressure, squeezing, or pain in the center of the chest, sometimes radiating to the shoulders, neck, jaw, arms, or upper back
- Shortness of breath
- Sweating
- Palpitations
- Fatigue

ATYPICAL SYMPTOMS
(WITH OR WITHOUT CHEST DISCOMFORT)
- Faintness or light-headedness
- Nausea or vomiting
- Fatigue

ELECTRICAL SYMPTOMS
(CAUSED BY DAMAGE TO THE HEART'S
ELECTRICAL SYSTEM)
- Irregular heartbeat
- Dizziness
- Racing, fast heartbeat (often perceived as palpitations)

SILENT SYMPTOMS
- None that you notice—that's why they're called silent!

It should be clear by now that you are playing Russian roulette with your health when you dismiss any symptoms as "no big deal." A small deal can turn into a big deal if it gets worse. If you notice chest pain that's getting more severe and takes less exertion to appear, or if you have increasing shortness of breath with less exercise, you need to see your doctor now. In tracking the missing half throughout this book, you'll see that missed warning signs account for a huge number of heart attacks that never make it into the emergency room.

STEP THREE:
DON'T WAIT!

Fatal Flaw

One of my parents' best friends developed sudden and unexpected chest pain at his home in suburban Boston. His wife's first instinct was to call the local hospital. Instead, she put him in her car and drove thirteen miles, in heavy traffic, to Massachusetts General Hospital in Boston. This is one of the best hospitals on the planet, but what a risk to take if you don't make it in time! Even after arriving at the hospital, rather than checking into the emergency department, she waited for his doctor to arrive. This is a textbook case of how to do everything the wrong way. If at any moment along the way he had suffered cardiac arrest, there was an extremely slim chance he would have survived.

During a heart attack, the biggest risk is what's euphemistically called "an electrical event." That's a wildly irregular heart rhythm called ventricular fibrillation, which means there is no effective pulse and no blood pressure, and there are just minutes before irreversible brain death occurs. It's irrecoverable without a defibrillator, and usually highly trained professionals who can administer cardiac drugs and other advanced treatments if defibrillation alone doesn't work. Every second you wait, you risk having your heart go into ventricular fibrillation. "If it does, the odds of survival drop by about 10 percent for each minute's delay in providing defibrillation. In other words, if your fibrillating heart can be 'shocked' with a defibrillator within three minutes, your chances of survival are roughly 70 percent. By five minutes, you're down to fifty–fifty. By ten minutes, you have only a one in ten chance of survival," says Dr. Joseph Ornato.

My parents' friend isn't alone. An astounding 50 percent of heart attack patients come in their own car, says Dr. Bruce MacLeod.

Conventional wisdom: It can wait.
The real deal: Don't be dead wrong.

Dick Cheney survived as long as he did by being extremely attentive to his heart symptoms. He was awakened at 3:30 A.M. by discomfort in his chest. Rather than dismissing it as indigestion, he headed to George Washington University Hospital. Even then, his condition was so subtle that the first lab tests and even the EKG showed nothing. By 7 A.M. his EKG showed minor abnormalities. He was moved to a catheterization suite where a 90 percent blockage was found in one of his arteries. He quickly underwent balloon therapy.

Don't wait. If you act in the first minutes, as Dick Cheney did, you may escape with no damage to your heart at all. Many of us wait, like ostriches, heads in the sand. This attitude is left over from the days when those symptoms heralded major damage to your heart or death, with little to be done but wait for the grim reaper.

This chapter puts together an action plan. Don't wait also applies to prevention. Start now and you may never have to call 911. This is a disease that waits for no one. The earlier you start, the better your chances. Remember, this is a recoverable disease. It's tragic but still understandable dying from an untreatable metastatic cancer. It's tragic but not understandable dying from an unforced error, which is what so many heart patients do. New medicines can prevent or limit damage from a heart attack, but they are most effective if given within an hour of the onset of symptoms. Tragically, data from the second National Registry of Myocardial Infarction ("myocardial infarction" is the medical term for heart attack) indicate that *only one in five patients gets to a hospital emergency department soon enough to benefit from these treatments.*

KNOW THE WARNING SIGNS

As soon as you notice any of the warning symptoms reviewed in the last chapter, you should spring into action. If you really believe you are having a heart attack, call 911. Be sure to use the words "chest pain" or "heart attack." If you already have heart disease or are at high risk, be sure to tell them that as well. This will put you at the top of the list of patients that the ambulances will rush to. Remember, if you have a sudden cardiac arrest, your chances of surviving drop 10 percent for every minute of delay until firefighters or paramedics can defibrillate you. Dr. James Atkins says, "The chance of resuscitation depends on many factors. In general, the chance of survival falls 10 percent per minute from the initial event. Since only a defibrillator can bring you back once you go into cardiac arrest, if you didn't call 911 prior to collapsing, you haven't got much of a chance (unless you're lucky enough to have a bystander recognize what's happened, call 911 immediately, and have a fire station with an available unit just around the corner). Your doctor may sound reassuring over the phone, but no cardiologist can reach through the phone line to save your life."

DON'T BE AFRAID OF SOUNDING DUMB

What if you think you're making a mistake and you're not suffering a heart attack? Far better wrong than dead. If trained emergency physicians can't tell for sure, you stand little chance of making the diagnosis on your own. Study after study shows that many patients are sent home from the hospital in error. Don't be afraid of erring on the side of caution.

Even cardiologists themselves can be as careless as the next person when they suffer symptoms of a heart attack. Here's Dr. Bruce McLeod's favorite story: "A really active cardiologist here had chest pain at a football game, and he said, 'I just had a hot dog.' So what did he do? He got another hot dog! Then he went home and said, 'Geez, it's going to my arm, what's going on? I must have pulled something or cheered too hard.' So he waited three hours before he came in, and he's having an acute MI. And this is a man who knows the most about what heart attack symptoms are."

What this story highlights is that even people who know better have a real sense of denial that anything bad can happen. Dr. MacLeod points out that 70 percent of heart attacks are not apparent on an EKG. It's only a series of blood tests over the course of the next eighteen hours that display the pattern characteristic of a heart attack. Commonly, an enzyme called creatine phosphokinase and a component of the contractile proteins of heart muscle called troponin slowly leak out of damaged heart muscle into the bloodstream. There is an MB fraction of CPK, which is more specific to heart muscle than skeletal muscle, to distinguish a heart attack from a bruised muscle in, say, your arm or leg.

CALL 911

This seems incredibly obvious, but the number one step that the majority of patients suffering heart attacks in the United States miss is calling 911. "The public uses paramedics when they have heart attack symptoms only about one in four times," says Dr. Joseph Ornato.

What do most patients do? They drive themselves to the hospital or have someone else drive them. The large NIH-sponsored REACT study revealed that only 23 percent of chest pain sufferers had called 911. About 60 percent were driven to the hospital by someone else. An astonishing 16 percent drove themselves to the hospital. If you call 911, you will get to the hospital much more quickly. Many have special tracing services that can find your home even if you're incapacitated halfway through the call and can no longer speak to 911.

Why do patients wait? They feel they are losing control. When they drive themselves, they delay, check the cat one last time, look for their purse or wallet, make a few phone calls, and second-guess their diagnosis. *Every* study shows that people who call 911 get to the hospital substantially earlier. Remember that time is your biggest enemy once your symptoms begin. How big a difference does time make? The MITI study in Seattle found that in patients treated within seventy minutes of the onset of their symptoms, less than 1 percent died. Few lost much heart muscle. Compare that to patients treated just one hour later. Twelve percent were dead at the end of the two-year study period.

CALL YOUR DOCTOR

Be sure to do this *after* you call the ambulance. Since you don't know if you may suddenly become incapacitated, you want 911 to know about you right away. Then call your doctor. While the ambulance is on its way, ask your doctor for specific instructions. Ask whether you should take an aspirin, take your nitroglycerin, or lie down. Have your doctor call the hospital you are going to and speak to the attending physician in the emergency department about important parts of your medical history and care, including key medications you are on. Your doctor may be able to meet the ambulance at the hospital. Give the ambulance driver your doctor's name once the driver knows which hospital you are going to. If your doctor knows that you are better off in another hospital, he or she can attempt to get involved in triage. For instance, you might need to be transferred to the best regional hospital for balloon therapy or bypass surgery.

GET THE RIGHT AMBULANCE

Calling 911 should mean that care arrives with the ambulance. Ambulances should no longer be a cart-and-carry service that just stuffs you in the back and transports you to care. The care should begin *in* the ambulance. But less than 20 percent of ambulance systems nationwide have sophisticated communications equipment that can send your EKG to the emergency department. Paramedics are highly skilled in the treatment of heart attack and can respond to physicians' orders from the emergency department to give you a wide variety of lifesaving medications, even clot-busting drugs, right in the ambulance. All this places you at the head of the line once you do reach the emergency department. Doctors and nurses know your up-to-the-minute status and stand by ready to treat you. If your condition is urgent, they can have balloon therapy treatment suite up and ready for you. If you had driven, you could wait for long periods in the emergency department before the urgency of your case became apparent.

Ambulances with EKGs on board can also get you to the right hospital. Doctors reading the EKG and talking with the paramedics can make a precise diagnosis and send you to a specialized cardiac unit. If you drive yourself to the local emergency department, it could well be the wrong one, without lifesaving drugs or balloon therapy. Since it's very hard and expensive to keep balloon therapy units up and on call twenty-four hours a day, one hospital in your area could be active during one eight-hour period and another during the next. Or one hospital could have suffered a power failure, or its intensive care unit might be full. Again, you could drive to what you think is the best hospital and end up waiting hours before you are transferred to the hospital with the active cardiac teams.

Cities like Dallas and Birmingham have up-to-date programs that inform the ambulances of the closest fully functioning and available cardiac center. There are areas in the United States that still do not have EKG- or defibrillator-equipped ambulances, resulting in a tragic loss of life. Check that the right ambulances are available in your area. Says Dr. James Atkins about the lack of availability of defibrillators in some communities: "It's a $20,000 machine that will last about seven years.

You've already paid $150,000 for an ambulance that will last two years, and you are paying $800,000 a year to staff it. That extra $20,000 is petty cash."

France is one of the few countries in the world that offer clot-busting drugs to heart attack patients before they reach the hospital. In the November 2003 issue of *Circulation,* the first randomized trial, based on the French experience, showed that clot-busting drugs seem preferable for patients treated within two hours of the onset of symptoms. Two to six hours after the event, patients do better with balloon therapy.

Philippe Gabriel Steg, M.D., director of the coronary care unit and an interventional cardiologist at Hôpital Bichat in Paris, says that France's compact size and highly urbanized population allow its emergency medical system to stabilize patients before transport to the nearest appropriate hospital. France also has mobile intensive care units staffed by doctors. These are sent to patients who call the French version of 911 complaining of chest pain.

Although the current American standard of care is the immediate use of balloon angioplasty after a heart attack, you should be aware of this study if you are offered clot busters in the ambulance, especially if you are a long distance from a hospital that offers balloon therapy.

HAVE A GAME PLAN

Carve out a half hour the next time you visit your cardiologist or internist. Get his or her input on a sensible 911 plan for you given your community's resources, its EMS system, and your insurer and your hospital's resources. Decide in advance which measures may make sense for you and which might be too risky if you do have a heart attack. Response time varies dramatically from one location to another, with the best response time in Seattle, and Washington, DC, near the bottom. Campaign for fast response times in your community. Tens of thousands of Americans die every year because ambulances get to them too late.

BE SURE YOU ARE AT THE RIGHT HOSPITAL

All hospitals are not created equal in terms of expertise and excellence. Many patients suffering a heart attack require balloon therapy. This is available only at a hospital with a highly specialized cardiac catheterization laboratory. In addition, the hospital should have the capability for backup bypass surgery. What's more, this therapy needs to be undertaken quickly, within 90 minutes of arrival. You have no time to waste. Often ambulances are directed to go to one specific hospital. This is dictated by space availability among other considerations.

To find the right hospital, you can look at its actual report card. The state peer review organization uses a very uniform abstraction method, so at least you are comparing apples to apples. For overall excellence in cardiology, see the list on pages 219–23 of the best hospitals for bypass surgery.

Do this research in advance and make it part of your game plan (pages 219–23). Then if you ever have to call 911, you can specify the hospital to which you want to go.

KNOW THE STANDARD OF CARE

You want to be very aware of exactly which treatment you should be receiving once you are in the ambulance and once you arrive in the ER. There is an established standard of care, which you should know. Below are descriptions of the medications and procedures that should be considered in your treatment before and after your arrival at the hospital. Don't expect to get all of these, but press for the right mixture of what's appropriate for what is happening to you. In one major study, an astounding 300 hospitals did not deliver the standard of care that is recommended at state-of-the-art centers. Even at some of the better hospitals, you may be at risk.

NITROGLYCERINE

When: immediately

Up to three nitroglycerine tablets may be taken for pain. In the ambulance, nitrous oxide or morphine may be given as well. It was once believed that relieving pain reduced the amount of damage done to the heart, but Dr. Joseph Ornato says that although nitroglycerine given during a heart attack may lessen the chest discomfort for a long time, randomized clinical trials have not shown that it lowers a heart attack victim's odds of dying.

Another bit of folklore: If nitroglycerine relieves the pain, it helps with the diagnosis. Joseph Ornato comments, "Wrong again. The response to nitroglycerine is as often misleading as helpful. This was an old clinical bit of folklore that hasn't held up. If you have pain, don't be afraid to ask for relief. You may be told no if you have low blood pressure, but there is no harm in asking." Dr. Jeffrey Borer adds that nitroglycerine is not itself a pain reliever, but it does improve the balance between heart muscle oxygen supply and demand, which in turn relieves pain.

The routine recommendation to use nitroglycerine is due to be changed in the American Heart Association's next series of recommendations. You can view them on the association's Web site at www.americanheart.org.

ASPIRIN

When: immediately

EXPERT COUNSEL

Dr. Joseph Ornato: "Take an aspirin as soon as possible. There had been some controversy following the initial GISSI 2 study, which showed benefit for ASA but no time dependence. Since then, the original data have been reanalyzed by the Israelis, and there appears to be a time relationship. That means it is urgent to take aspirin as soon as possible after the onset of a heart attack, at the direction of your doctor or paramedics. It will lower your chances of dying from a heart attack, *but it will not take the heart attack away,* so do not take aspirin and 'wait for it to work' instead of calling 911 promptly. Such a mistake could cost your life."

EXPERT COUNSEL

Dr. James Atkins: "Most of us say take an aspirin immediately."

An aspirin may be taken once a heart attack is suspected as long as you have no history of aspirin allergy. Says James Atkins, "I know very little harm of aspirin, so in our ambulances in Dallas, everyone gets an aspirin."

I asked Jeffrey Borer if you should take aspirin if you are already on daily aspirin. "Yes. It doesn't matter if the patient is already taking aspirin. You don't know how much the patient has taken, you don't know if it's been absorbed, etc. I suggest a chewable aspirin; it's certainly safe for the vast majority of people." There is an acute inflammatory component of an acute heart attack, and to the degree that aspirin has an effect on that, there's an urgency to taking aspirin.

CLOPIDOGREL (PLAVIX)

The blood thinner clopidogrel, when used with aspirin, reduces the risk of subsequent heart attack, stroke, and death in people who come to the ER with new or increasing chest pain or heart attack, as reported in the journal *Circulation*. Dr. Jeffrey Borer adds that data from the CURE trial now suggest that clopidogrel with aspirin does better than aspirin alone.

This super new drug is described in full in Step 6, "Take Lifesaving Medications." Clopidogrel is usually given to patients with unstable chest pain and heart attack patients who do not have the typical EKG changes. The earlier the better is the watchword, although convincing research data are not complete.

The catch is that clopidogrel shouldn't be given to a patient who may need bypass surgery, because it substantially increases the risk of bleeding. If you go to the cath lab for immediate balloon therapy, you'll get clopidogrel started once it is clear that you can be treated adequately without an immediate trip to the operating room for bypass surgery.

STATINS

When: within 24 hours

These are cholesterol-lowering superdrugs about which there is a large section in Step 6.

Data suggest that taking statins very early in the course of a heart attack or acute coronary syndrome may reduce your chance of dying. Statins have a powerful and fast effect on blockages. They also improve the function of endothelial cells that line the coronary arteries. They do this by altering nitric oxide synthase activity, benefiting the release of nitric oxide, which directly dilates the coronary arteries, improving blood flow. And of course statins lower levels of inflammation in coronary arteries.

EXPERT COUNSEL
Dr. James Atkins: "You want to take a statin very early on. Again, this is something for which we don't know all of the answers because we always thought the only way statins were working was by lowering LDL cholesterol. We now recognize the inflammatory component."

BETA-BLOCKERS

When: within 24 hours

Beta-blockers reduce the heart's oxygen requirement and, thus, the size of the heart attack, counsels Dr. Joseph Ornato. "Longer term, they reduce the risk of sudden death, especially in patients with anterior wall and/or large heart attacks." Says Dr. James Atkins, "There is benefit of beta-blockers at any time as long as they are tolerated; however, the sooner the better. There is evidence that giving beta-blockers in the first hour is very important. There were studies done many years ago with metoprolol in Europe. They gave patients IV metoprolol [e.g., Lopressor] when they hit the emergency department door, and there was a survival benefit. Metoprolol needs to be continuously given and, for many people, very early."

Beta-blockers also block adrenaline. During a heart attack, your body produces extra adrenaline, which makes platelets stickier, which in turn makes it easier for artery-blocking blood cells to form.

Unfortunately, with all the benefits, your chances of getting a beta-blocker depend very much on where you live. Beta-blockers are very highly used in the Northeast, moderately heavily used in Texas, very seldom used in Kansas. There are national guidelines, but many parts of the country don't follow them as much as they should. Dr. Bruce McLeod says it's one of the most common mistakes in treatment, and he is concerned that many heart attack patients are not given beta-blockers early and are not discharged on beta-blockers.

GLYCOPROTEIN IIB/IIIA

When: immediately

These are used only in specific situations. They require your doctor to be specific about what he or she sees on the EKG.

If you have unstable angina but not a heart attack, or if you have a heart attack that does not show what is termed ST elevation on the EKG, then glycoprotein IIb/IIIa may be helpful. With a larger heart attack, the goal is to dissolve or remove a clot, which is when clot busters come into play. In this situation, however, you have a clot that's layered in but not blocking the vessel, so you want to keep it from propagating. Glycoprotein IIb/IIIa can accomplish this, says Dr. James Atkins. The same is true of heparin.

Dr. Joseph Ornato also recommends glycoprotein IIb/IIIa for heart attack patients with ST elevation on the EKG who are going to the cath lab or having a balloon angioplasty.

ACE INHIBITORS

When: within 24 hours

ACE inhibitors may play a large role in the ultimate performance of your heart after a heart attack, especially if your heart is pumping poorly and has a low ejection fraction, meaning that it is pumping much less blood per heartbeat than it should.

ACE inhibitors remodel the heart's main pumping chamber, the left ventricle. The heart normally is elliptical, but when there's a heart attack, it becomes round. ACE inhibitors inhibit it from becoming more round or even return it to a more elliptical shape. This makes the heart much more efficient at pumping and may help prevent heart failure. (ACE inhibitors are described in full in Step 6.)

CLOT-BUSTING DRUGS (THROMBOLYTICS)

When: 30 minutes or less after hospital arrival

Since the damage from a heart attack begins when a blood clot closes a coronary artery, the goal is to dissolve the clot and restore the flow of blood as quickly as possible. Because there is some risk involved, and since there are other techniques to open your coronary artery, doctors weigh this decision very judiciously. Some paramedics have been authorized to use clot-busting drugs in the ambulance. They decide by observing an ST elevation on your EKG, which is highly indicative of a heart attack.

Time is supercritical at this point—with every hour that goes by, your odds of death increase. The best time to minimize your chance of heart muscle damage and death is in the first 60 to 90 minutes. During that time, the goal is to open the artery that has closed and is causing your heart attack. This can be accomplished with a clot-busting drug, balloon therapy, or even bypass surgery. One of the best studies is the MITI, which showed that patients who got the clot-busting drug TPA in the first 70 minutes after onset of symptoms did significantly better. Whether it was given by paramedics in the ambulance or by doctors in the emergency department didn't matter, just the elapsed time. The death rate was only 2 percent when given in the first 70 minutes. However, in the next time block, 70 to 180 minutes, the death rate quadrupled to 8 percent.

So time really does make a highly critical difference for heart attacks. Can you add aspirin to clot busters? There is a theory that aspirin given with the clot-busting drug streptokinase may help to open an artery sooner. At present, cardiologists believe that mechanically clearing or bypassing the blockage yields better results than clot busters in patients who are a good risk. For the procedure, the most recent studies show a clear superiority in lives saved by using balloon therapy over clot-busting drugs. If balloon therapy is not available, or you are not eligible, the clot-busting drugs are the next best treatment.

If you and your doctor decide that you are not a candidate for clot-busting drugs, be sure that you are headed toward a hospital that offers balloon therapy and bypass surgery.

WHICH KIND OF CLOT BUSTER IS BEST?

Two key clot busters, the more expensive alteplase or TPA (tissue plasminogen activator) and the less expensive streptokinase, have been tested head to head. The GUSTO-1 study showed clear superiority of TPA over streptokinase, concludes Dr. Joseph Ornato. TPA is 10 percent better than streptokinase when you are looking at mortality and morbidity. Here is a complete list of the available clot busters:

- alteplase, TPA (Activase)
- anistreplase (Eminase)

- lanoteplase
- reteplase (Retavase)
- staphylokinase (STAR)
- streptokinase (Streptase)
- tenecteplase (TNKase)
- urokinase (Abbokinase)

ANTIDEPRESSANTS

A recent study in *Circulation* reported that treating depression in heart attack or chest pain patients reduces the chances of forming dangerous new blood clots. "This study is the first to show that the antidepressant sertraline [Zoloft] inhibits platelet endothelial markers more than placebo in depressed patients after coronary events," says lead author Dr. Victor L. Serebruany, assistant professor of medicine at Johns Hopkins University and laboratory director for Sinai Thrombosis Center in Baltimore.

"In depressed patients," the study continues, "platelets in the blood are stickier and more likely to form clots. Previous studies have shown that depressed patients are more likely than non-depressed patients to die of a subsequent cardiac problem after being hospitalized for a heart attack. After a heart attack, 20 percent to 25 percent of patients develop major depression, but it often goes untreated."

Some cardiologists feel a real sense of urgency to begin antidepressant therapy in the cardiac care unit.

ANGIOGRAM

When: 90 minutes or less after hospital arrival
Once doctors see on your EKG that you are suffering a heart attack and have looked at other confirmatory tests, they need to

know its precise location and if it is feasible physically to remove or bypass the blockage in your artery that is causing your heart attack. An angiogram allows them to see the blockage and decide on further therapy, which may include balloon therapy or bypass surgery. In order for this to happen, you must be in a hospital that has an active and operating angiogram suite at the time you arrive.

BALLOON THERAPY

When: 90 minutes or less after hospital arrival

If doctors find a blockage in your coronary artery, they may be able to push the blood clot aside, open up the vessel, and insert a stent, sparing a good deal of your heart muscle from dying. They should discuss carefully with you the difficulty of approaching your blockage and the risk involved. At present, balloon therapy is favored over bypass surgery and clot-busting drugs.

BYPASS SURGERY

When: 90 minutes or less after hospital arrival

If you have a very difficult to approach blockage, your doctor may consider bypass surgery. This is especially true if your blockage is in a very dangerous place, such as the beginning of the left anterior descending coronary artery. Step 7, "Get the Right Lifesaving Procedure," describes bypass surgery in detail.

PREVENTION

There is a major shift from secondary prevention to primary prevention. Hundreds of thousands of Americans begin their prevention program after their first heart attack. You don't want to wait to start cholesterol-lowering or inflammation-damping therapy until after a bad event has occurred. By the time you have a first heart attack, at least one of your heart's arteries has already narrowed by at least 75 percent. Remember that heart disease is rarely genetic, occurring genetically in only about one person in 500.

For decades doctors have been satisfied with slowing the progress of the disease, which only delays the inevitable. The new goal is to prevent heart disease entirely and arrest or even reverse the formation of plaques in your arteries. Is that possible? Remember that the chances of plaque formation are small if your total cholesterol is 150 mg/dL and your LDL cholesterol is below 100 mg/dL. Although there is huge rush to use balloon therapy, stents, and pacemakers and defibrillators, there's much less will to spend the time, money, and resources necessary to prevent the disease. This chapter is the most critical in the book in the event you do have a heart attack sometime in the future.

You don't have to remember a lot. These simple points will help you get the right treatment in time to save your life or that of a loved one. Most of the missing half did wait too long. Don't be one of them.

STEP FOUR: DETERMINE YOUR RISK

> ### Fatal Flaw
>
> "My cholesterol is great," Janice bragged to her office-mates. And it was—just above "normal." A week later she was dead of a fatal heart attack. How could a test have been so wrong?
>
> Janice had her cholesterol measured at a health fair. The technicians measured only her total cholesterol. By failing to perform a more complete test, the lab technicians missed a frighteningly low good HDL cholesterol; it was far too low to protect her. Even worse, they missed an even more dangerously high level of bad LDL cholesterol. Adding to the lethal mix, Janice had slightly elevated blood sugar, enough to make her diabetic, though she never knew. Her doctor brushed off her tests, calling them "pretty normal."
>
> Like millions of Americans, Janice had simply failed to get the right tests and the right interpretation. Worse still,

her strong family history should have tipped off her doctor. She should have had a complete cholesterol panel. This would have alerted any good cardiologist and led to much more vigorous testing and treatment. Getting a CRP to test for inflammation was never considered. She joined the silent half of patients whose first sign of heart disease is sudden death.

Conventional wisdom: My test scores are perfect.
The real deal: Don't count on incomplete results.

Your coronary arteries may be lined with dozens of plaques, any one of which could fracture at any given moment. Clearly, the best strategy of all is to defuse these potential time bombs with intensive medical therapy. Is this something you really need to do? You'll know only by determining your personal risk.

GET THE RIGHT TESTS

The right tests can tip you off years to decades before you suffer a heart attack. They're often simple and cheap, but most of us never get them. This chapter and the next will help you pick your way through the high-technology choices. There are two kinds of tests:

- Tests that look for causes of heart disease but don't look for the disease itself. These are risk factors such as high cholesterol, high blood pressure, or inflammation. These tests are described in this chapter.

- Tests that look for the disease itself, such as real structural problems with your heart, from weak heart muscle to blocked arteries. As these tests increase in precision, there is an additional risk. Many are high-tech marvels that can pinpoint precisely where trouble lies. Your doctor will order these based on troubling symptoms, high risk, and alarming blood tests. There is a logical progression. Without risk factors or symptoms, there is usually no need for more testing. With risk factors, safe and inexpensive tests are usually performed first. More sophisticated and riskier tests are undertaken only as a prelude to balloon therapy or surgery. These are described in Step 5, "Get the Right Diagnosis."

TESTS THAT LOOK FOR CAUSES

HSCRP

High sensitivity C-reactive protein (hsCRP) is the biggest and most important new risk factor. It indicates inflammation in the plaques lining your heart's arteries. The fundamental thinking is that atherosclerosis is an inflammatory disease just like arthritis. CRP, when measured with new high-sensitivity tests, is a strong predictor of who will have a stroke or a heart attack— even when cholesterol levels are *low*. Remember that half of all heart attacks occur in people like Janice who have average cholesterol levels. The best news is that if you do have a high hsCRP, you can easily reduce it. Moreover, as Dr. Paul Ridker tell us, evidence is rapidly accumulating that CRP is not just a marker of disease but also plays a major role in the disease process itself.

What's more, CRP is a great predictor of adult-onset diabetes, warning you years in advance that you may be on your way to real trouble. How does all this hang together? Inflammation is a key component of many of the biggest killers. The reason is interesting. During millions of years of human evolution, people with enhanced inflammatory systems survived. In the survival of the fittest, they were the most fit because their bodies could fight infection better. But now that antibiotics have largely eliminated infection as a cause of death, many of us are left with overactive inflammatory systems that attack our own bodies with a vengeance.

The good news is that statins, the same drugs that lower your cholesterol, also lower your CRP. Even better, if you have high cholesterol and high CRP, statins work more powerfully, significantly reducing your risk of heart disease. Dr. Paul Ridker states that "statins lower both LDL cholesterol and CRP levels and they appear to be more affective in terms of preventing heart attacks when the CRP levels are high." This means that the statins lower both LDL and CRP, which is extremely important.

Aspirin also works to reduce the risk of heart disease even in patients with a high CRP. Dr. Ridker reports that his team "showed back in 1996 that aspirin, a very commonly used drug to prevent first-ever heart attacks, works better in the presence of a high CRP than a low CRP. That's exciting if you think about it because aspirin is an anti-inflammatory drug, so this marker of inflammation tells us something about how the drug works."

You can see there are a variety of really good reasons for you to lower your CRP and easy ways to do it as well. It's one test you should insist getting. It costs about $20 and can be ordered at the same time as your cholesterol test.

What remains controversial is whether or not people with low cholesterol levels but high levels of hsCRP should be treated with statins. Dr. Ridker is careful to point out that we don't yet have evidence that lowering CRP levels necessarily lowers cardiac risk. So he and his group have organized a major national trial of randomized patients with low cholesterol levels who also have high levels of hsCRP to see if statins help prevent first heart attacks and strokes.

TAKING THE TEST

An elevated hsCRP does not automatically mean you are at high risk of heart disease. Recent colds, flu, and arthritis can all elevate CRP, even if you have no heart disease. Dr. Roger Blumenthal, associate professor of medicine in the Division of Cardiology at Johns Hopkins, suggests having two tests, two months apart, and averaging the results. "And if a level appeared very high ($\geq$ 10 mg/L), your doctor should search for an obvious source of infection or inflammation, which could obscure any prediction of coronary risk that might be attributed to the elevated level. That large result should then be discarded and the hsCRP measured again in two weeks."

Recent data from Paul Ridker's group suggests, however, that your risk may well be very high if your hsCRP is consistently above 10 mg/L. This suggests that almost any source of chronic inflammation is bad, at least from your heart's perspective.

WHO SHOULD GET TESTED

Every adult. The hsCRP test should be taken along with your cholesterol panel because the two tests identify different risks. Half of the people who develop heart disease have normal cholesterol levels. A CRP test can also serve as a tiebreaker when considering drug treatment to reduce risk factors. This is most important for those with "intermediate" levels of LDL cholesterol between 130 and 160 mg/dL where elevated hsCRP might well lead your doctor to prescribe a statin.

CHOLESTEROL

When cholesterol first became a media superstar, knowing your "cholesterol number" alone was considered pretty sophisticated. Now the standard is a panel of tests, which include total cholesterol, HDL cholesterol, and triglyceride measurement. From those measurements, the lab technician will calculate your LDL or bad cholesterol. The official recommendations just ten years ago suggested only an initial total cholesterol and perhaps an HDL. Today, according to Dr. Luther Clark, it is suggested that you get a full lipid profile, rather than screening for total cholesterol and HDL alone.

WHO SHOULD GET TESTED

The top experts believe that everyone over twenty should know his or her lipid profile. The frequency of testing depends on your results. Says Dr. Steven Nissen, "People aren't checking cholesterol until they get into their middle-aged years because all the studies have focused on individuals forty, fifty, and on up. But many of us have made the argument that disease prevention starts much earlier in life. Therefore, one has to think a little more proactively about intercepting the disease before it's so extensive."

TAKING THE TEST

Fast for at least twelve hours before the test. Water is permissible.

Dr. Steven Nissen comments on an aspect of human nature: "There's a funny thing that people sometimes do. When people know they are going to get their cholesterol checked next week, they sometimes alter their diet before the test. You really ought to go on eating your customary diet."

UNDERSTANDING YOUR TEST RESULTS

The National Cholesterol Education Program from the NHLBI has set tough new cutoff points that reflect increased knowledge about the relationship between a low HDL and an increased risk of heart disease and about the dangers of moderate LDL for those already at risk. Check your results against the values below.

TOTAL CHOLESTEROL
- < 200: Desirable
- 200–239: Borderline high
- ≥ 240: High

LDL
The new LDL guidelines identify an optimal level of < 100 mg/dL as opposed to the old guidelines of < 130 mg/dL.

- < 100: Optimal
- 100–129: Near optimal/above optimal. If you have other risk factors, then your LDL should be below 130, and that's without any marked symptoms, cardiac history, or major risk factors. One risk factor is age alone, males above forty-five, women above fifty-five.
- 130–159: Borderline high
- 160–189: High
- ≥ 190: Very high

HDL
Low HDL is emerging as a powerhouse new risk factor for heart disease. Doctors used to view high HDL as a major plus, but they didn't rate the downside of low HDL. Since this is your body's internal artery-cleaning solution, like a chemical Roto-

Rooter, too little can really hurt you. The old cutoff point was 35. The new cutoff point is 40.

- < 10 mg/dL: Low. You are at risk for heart disease.
- > 60 mg/dL: Very high. This confers strong protection. My mother, who is ninety, has HDL near 90.

EXPERT ADVICE

Dr. Steven Nissen: "Most patients ask about their total cholesterol, but that number alone really doesn't tell us much. I think people ought to be more sophisticated and know what their 'bad' and 'good' cholesterol levels are. Often when I ask patients if they've had their cholesterol checked, they say, 'Yes, my family doctor checked it.' When I ask what it was, they say, 'My total cholesterol was under 200. I'm okay, right?' "

Dr. Nissen points out that they may not be okay. Take the example of Janice, the undiagnosed diabetic whose cholesterol was 200. Pretty good value, you might say, even below average. But she was a ticking time bomb.

Let's say your total cholesterol is 200, your bad cholesterol is 160, your good cholesterol is 20, and your triglycerides are 100.

$$\text{total cholesterol} = \text{HDL} + \text{LDL} + (\text{triglycerides} \div 5)$$

This gives you a total of 20 + 160 + 20 = 200. Sure, the total cholesterol looks fine—until you realize that it's nearly *all* bad cholesterol. At 160, your LDL cholesterol is considered high even though your total cholesterol is normal. "It's time for the public to understand the numbers, because their doctors may not," concludes Dr. Nissen. Claude Lenfant agrees: "Know your numbers."

TRIGLYCERIDES

Experts are placing greater emphasis on elevated triglycerides as a marker for increased risk for chronic heart disease. Don't be surprised if in addition to an elevated triglyceride level, you have other lipid problems. Elevated triglycerides are commonly associated with lipid and nonlipid risk factors. Causes of elevated triglycerides include obesity, lack of exercise, smoking, excess alcohol intake, high-carbohydrate diets, diabetes, metabolic syndrome, and genetic predisposition. Also note that triglycerides and HDL tend to go in opposite directions. That is, you'll have high triglycerides and low HDL, or vice versa.

Compare the results on your laboratory report with the values below.

- < 150 mg/dL: Normal
- 150–199 mg/dL: Borderline-high
- 200–499 mg/dL: High
- ≥ 500 mg/dL: Very high

First-line therapy for elevated triglycerides is lifestyle changes: lose weight, exercise, stop smoking, cut down on alcohol and carbohydrates. There are also specific triglyceride-lowering medications, which include the following. (Step 6, "Take Lifesaving Medications," has much more detail.)

- Nicotinic acid
- Fibric acid derivatives
- Statins
- Cholesterol absorption inhibitors

- Bile acid sequestrants
- N-3 omega fatty acids

What to do next? Your primary care physician can arrange for cholesterol tests. But what if the results are difficult to interpret or they have what Steven Nissen calls "very unusual, oddball abnormalities, let's say the triglycerides are in the thousands or you've had toxicity from drugs"? Then you should see a specialist.

FASTING BLOOD SUGAR

More than 13 million Americans have been diagnosed, and it is estimated that 5 million more are diabetic but don't know it. This means that everyone—even children—should probably be tested. The simplest first-line screening test is the measurement of your blood sugar level after fasting overnight. If you are even mildly over the limit, your risk of heart disease climbs steeply. The test costs about $15.

TAKING THE TEST

Do not eat or drink anything except water after about 10 P.M. the night before the test. A technician will draw one small tube of blood from your arm.

TEST RESULTS

Your fasting blood sugar should be less than 110. The American Diabetes Association may soon recommend dropping the maximum to 100.

GLUCOSE TOLERANCE TEST

A much more sensitive test is a glucose tolerance test. You will be given a large amount of glucose (a form of sugar) to drink. Two hours later, your blood sugar will be measured. The norm for a two-hour glucose is less than 140. If your two-hour glucose remains between 140 and 199, you are at high risk for type 2 diabetes. This also puts you at greater risk for coronary artery disease.

NEW RISK FACTORS

Kidney specialists have long known that patients on dialysis with late-stage kidney disease have a ten- to thirtyfold greater risk than the general population of dying of cardiovascular events such as a heart attack or heart failure. The American Heart Association in a recent statement in *Circulation* placed people with chronic kidney disease, even those in the early stages of the disorder, in the highest risk group for cardiovascular disease.

OPTIONAL TESTS

These specific tests are for what are termed "emerging risk factors," which are aimed at finding subclinical disease, that is, disease without signs or symptoms. Remember that doctors fail to predict as many as half of heart attacks based on cholesterol testing alone. That's why you may want to consider further testing.

How do you and your doctor decide how aggressive your treatment should be? There are several tiebreakers that may help you decide if you're on the fence. If the results of these tests are strongly positive, you ought to press for very aggressive therapy. Two prime candidates are those with a strong family history of heart disease and those with metabolic syndrome. In both circumstances, your other screening tests may not be alarming at all, so you could easily end up undertreated. Why? The Framingham score does not account for family history, and the national treatment guidelines don't account for either family history or metabolic syndrome. The true risk in persons with a first-degree relative with early heart disease is two to three times higher.

This allows millions of patients to fall through the cracks, accounting for tens of thousands of deaths each year, just like Janice. If these tiebreakers are strongly positive, press for aggressive treatment even if you don't fall under the guidelines. As Dr. Steven Nissen says, "These tiebreakers are for someone who doesn't quite make it on the Framingham score but the doctor thinks he or she may really have heart disease. These push you over the brink toward treating them."

If your doctor is reluctant to provide more aggressive treatment, go elsewhere, ideally a large center of excellence in heart disease or a major center that has a specialized lipid center.

LP(A)

Lp(a) is a lipoprotein found in LDL. Studies have found a correlation between high levels of Lp(a) and heart disease and stroke. A recent study in *Circulation* indicates that apolipoprotein B (apoB), a component of Lp(a) may be a better predictor of cardiovascular disease risk. Lp(a) may promote blood clotting and worsen inflammation.

EXPERT ADVICE

Dr. Richard Stein: "I test for Lp(a) in patients who have coronary disease with no other risk factor; say, young people with heart attacks and stroke. I also look for it in anyone with a significant family history. Increasingly I'm doing Lp(a)s in patients who have coronary disease because it gives me a marker as to how low to lower their other risk factors. I'd be more aggressive in the presence of Lp(a). I don't do it as part of a routine screen unless there's a family history."

EXPERT COUNSEL

Dr. Christie Ballantyne, Department of Medicine at Baylor College of Medicine: "Measuring Lp(a) is particularly useful if you have a family history of coronary disease, because it's genetic. So if you've got a bad family history, you might want to look into having an Lp(a) measurement."

EXPERT DISSENT

Dr. Steven Nissen: "Many of us think this is a waste of money. If you have high triglycerides, you almost always have small dense LDL particles."

TREATMENT FOR HIGH LP(A)

Lp(a) can be lowered by niacin. The alternative approach is to try to lower LDL cholesterol more aggressively with a statin and other therapies.

Says Dr. Christie Ballantyne, "Statins are the first approach to reducing the number of 'bad' particles, and combination therapy with ezetimibe (Zetia)—a cholesterol absorption inhibitor—or with a bile acid–binding resin can provide greater reductions. Niacin and fibrates (fenofibrate and gemfibrozil) raise HDL and also favorably change particle size."

HOMOCYSTEINE

High homocysteine levels were, for a few years, the most promising new explanation for otherwise unexplained heart attacks. Too much of this amino acid may irritate and damage the arteries, increasing the possibility of blood clots. However, the link between high homocysteine and heart disease has not been proved beyond a shadow of a doubt; the risk of heart disease may not be that high even if your level is elevated. If you have unexplained heart disease or are at high risk, you could consider this test, which costs $75 to $150.

TAKING THE TEST

A blood sample is taken from a vein, and either plasma or serum is tested.

UNDERSTANDING YOUR TEST RESULTS

Dr. Donald Jacobsen, director of the Laboratory for Homocysteine Research at the Cleveland Clinic Foundation, offers some guidelines. "Each lab has its own 'normal range.' The upper limit of normal thus varies somewhat from lab to lab. Making things even more complicated is the fact that premenopausal women's homocysteine levels are approximately 20 percent lower than those of their male counterparts. Also, homocysteine levels increase with age. Eventually we will use age-gender-dependent upper limits of normal, but this is generally not the case now. To grossly simplify the matter, use an upper limit of normal of 10 micromolar (plasma) for middle-aged adults. If a serum sample is analyzed, the upper limit of normal is 12 micromolar."

Taking folate and vitamins B_6 and B_{12} makes good sense if your homocysteine level is elevated.

SMOKING

This risk factor does not require a test—you know if you smoke. Smoking is one of the greatest risk factors for heart disease. Even twenty years ago, at the Peter Bent Brigham, heart attacks in men in their fifties and women in their sixties were fairly uncommon if they did not smoke. Smoking is a lethal accelerator of coronary artery disease.

WHAT IS YOUR RISK?

Now that you know your basic laboratory values, you can put them all together with the following risk assessment. A big part of deciding how vigorously you should pursue testing and treatment depends on your risk. Remember that a moderate to high risk can tip you off years before you suffer the first symptoms of disease. The tables below include everything but family history and CRP. You can assume that if you have family history of heart disease, your risk is double.

This is a simplified coronary prediction test that you can

take yourself, based on the blood pressure, total cholesterol, and LDL categories proposed by the fifth Joint National Committee report on the detection, evaluation, and treatment of high blood pressure and the National Cholesterol Education Programs.

Estimate your risk for heart disease over the next ten years, based on the Framingham study of men and women thirty to seventy-four years old at baseline. The Framingham study is the longest continuous observation of men, women, and children and the subsequent appearance of heart disease. Select the value on the left that best describes you and circle the number of points on the right. Add up your total points at the end to determine your risk. There are separate tests for men and women.

RISK ASSESSMENT FOR MEN

Step 1: Age alone is a major risk factor: The older you are, the higher your risk. Being sixty years old puts you at the same risk as having total cholesterol over 280 and LDL over 190, the top scores in this test.

AGE

Years	Points
30–34	−1
35–39	0
40–44	1
45–49	2
50–54	3
55–59	4
60–64	5
65–69	6
70–74	7

Step 2: Select your LDL cholesterol.

LDL CHOLESTEROL	
mg/dL	Points
< 100	–3
100–129	0
130–159	0
160–190	1
≥ 190	2

Step 3: Select your HDL cholesterol.

HDL CHOLESTEROL	
mg/dL	Points
< 35	2
35–44	1
45–49	0
50–59	0
≥ 60	–1

Step 4: Select your systolic blood pressure in the column on the left and then your diastolic blood pressure in the horizontal row. Where they intersect is your score.

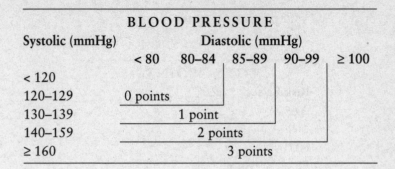

BLOOD PRESSURE

Systolic (mmHg)   Diastolic (mmHg)

	< 80	80–84	85–89	90–99	≥ 100
< 120					
120–129	0 points				
130–139		1 point			
140–159			2 points		
≥ 160			3 points		

Step 5

DIABETES

	Points
No	0
Yes	2

Step 6

SMOKER

	Points
No	0
Yes	2

Step 7: Add your points from steps 1–6.

TOTAL POINTS

Risk Factor	Points
Age	
LDL	
HDL	
Blood pressure	
Diabetes	
Smoker	
Total points	

Step 8: Find your total score on the left and your ten-year risk on the right.

CORONARY ARTERY DISEASE RISK

Total Points	Ten-Year Risk
< –3	1%
–2	2%
–1	2%
0	3%
1	4%
2	4%
3	6%
4	7%
5	9%
6	11%
7	14%
8	18%
9	22%
10	27%

11	33%
12	40%
13	47%
≥ 14	≥ 56%

- Greater than 20% risk in ten years is very high.
- Between 10–20% is moderately high.
- Less than 10% is low.

Step 9: Finally, compare your risk to that of the general population in your age group.

COMPARATIVE RISK

Age	Average Ten-Year Risk
30–34	< 1%
35–39	< 1%
40–44	2%
45–49	5%
50–54	8%
55–59	12%
60–64	12%
65–69	13%
70–74	14%

RISK ASSESSMENT FOR WOMEN

Select the value on the left that best describes you and circle the number of points on the right. Your total points signify your risk.

Step 1: Age alone is a major risk factor: The older you are, the higher your risk. Being sixty years old puts you at the same risk as having total cholesterol over 280 and LDL over 190, the top scores in this test.

AGE	
Years	Points
30–34	–9
35–39	–4
40–44	0
45–49	3
50–54	6
55–59	7
60–64	8
65–69	8
70–74	8

Step 2: Find your LDL cholesterol.

LDL CHOLESTEROL	
mg/dL	Points
< 100	–2
100–129	0
130–159	0
160–190	2
≥ 190	2

Step 3: Find your HDL cholesterol.

HDL CHOLESTEROL	
mg/dL	Points
< 35	5
35–44	2
45–49	1
50–59	0
≥ 60	–2

Step 4: Select your systolic blood pressure in the column on the left and then your diastolic blood pressure in the horizontal row. Where they intersect is your score.

BLOOD PRESSURE

Systolic mmHg	Diastolic (mmHg)				
	< 80	80–84	85–89	90–99	≥ 100
< 120	–3 points				
120–129	0 points				
130–139					
140–159	2 points				
≥ 160	3 points				

Step 5

DIABETES	
	Points
No	0
Yes	4

Step 6

SMOKER

	Points
No	0
Yes	2

Step 7: Add your points from steps 1–6.

TOTAL POINTS

Risk factor	Points
Age	
LDL	
HDL	
Blood pressure	
Diabetes	
Smoker	
Total points	

Step 8: Find your total score on the left and your ten-year risk on the right.

CORONARY ARTERY DISEASE RISK

Total Points	Ten-Year Risk
< –2	1%
–1	2%
0	2%
1	2%
2	3%
3	3%

4	4%
5	5%
6	6%
7	7%
8	8%
9	9%
10	11%
11	13%
12	15%
13	17%
14	20%
15	24%
16	27%
≥ 17	≥ 32%

Step 9: Finally, compare your risk to that of the general population in your age group.

COMPARATIVE RISK

Age	Average Ten-Year Risk
30–34	< 1%
35–39	< 1%
40–44	2%
45–49	5%
50–54	8%
55–59	12%
60–64	12%
65–69	13%
70–74	14%

The most practical use of these tests is to indicate how aggressive your medical therapy should be and whether you should consider the screening tests in the following chapter. According to Dr. Roger Blumenthal, if you are asymptomatic but have a greater than 10 percent risk of heart attack over the next ten years, then you should get your LDL down to less than 130. If you have a greater than 20 percent risk over the next ten years, your target LDL should be less than 100.

THE BIG PICTURE

Look at your whole package with your physician, including your family history and physical exam. Don't focus on just one test. As we saw with Janice, you could easily get a series of screening tests and miss the big picture. For instance, you could have mild elevations of cholesterol, blood pressure, and blood sugar, but your doctor misses the diagnosis of metabolic syndrome, a huge risk factor. This is one of the largest groups that are not yet recognized or brought into treatment, says Dr. Luther Clark. If your cholesterol is mildly elevated and you are even slightly diabetic, you have a huge risk of heart disease. You could become part of the missing half.

Many physicians may reassure you and say you don't need to worry, but in fact you need to worry a lot, until you get your risk factors under control. As I've stressed throughout this book, multiple minor abnormalities can be significant. Also remember inflammation. An elevated hsCRP predicts increased risk at all levels of the Framingham Risk Score, at all levels of LDL cholesterol, and at all levels of metabolic syndrome.

STEP FIVE: GET THE RIGHT DIAGNOSIS

THE last chapter looked at pure risk, those factors like choles-terol, inflammation, and high blood pressure that can cause heart disease but by no means prove you have it. This chapter looks at precise tests that pinpoint actual structural or func-tional abnormalities of the heart.

There is often a progression to these tests, beginning with those that could cause little harm to those that involve some risk. In addition, doctors test for the most common problems first.

TESTS THAT LOOK FOR DISEASE

CALCIUM SCAN/ ELECTRON-BEAM TOMOGRAPHY (EBT)/MULTIDETECTOR CT

Cost: $400–$500

The buzzword in modern cardiology is "subclinical" dis-ease. That means finding disease before you have symptoms.

Many of the missing half I've looked at in this book had subclinical disease that didn't produce any symptoms. Autopsies of children killed in accidents or young soldiers killed in combat both show extensive "streaking" in coronary arteries. There are already fatty deposits as early as grade school, leading to the conclusion that coronary artery disease is a disease of childhood that shows up in middle age. You've learned about tests that detect risk factors, which can warn you about early disease, but is there an actual test to find early disease?

Yes. Electron-beam tomography operates under the theory that as cholesterol blockages grow and age in coronary arteries, they become calcified, and that calcium should show up on a scan. The latest version, called 16-slice, has some of the abilities of an intravascular ultrasound to look inside blood vessel walls. But in contrast to the intravascular ultrasound, a catheter doesn't need to be threaded into your heart. The EBT is completely noninvasive.

Sounds good. So why is there so much controversy—and even hostility—about this test? Many cardiologists are angry about the calcium scan and see it as big waste of money. You can order an EBT without a doctor's referral, and it has become a huge revenue generator. Dr. Steven Nissen says that in California, for example, "You can go to the local mall to get a calcium scan. They advertise on the radio, they have billboards. 'Buy your honey a CT scan for Valentine's Day.'" Why the uproar over consumers plunking down their own hard-earned cash for this test?

Here's the problem as put forward by the critics. Sure, you could have calcium in your coronaries, but it may pose no risk. Or if it does pose a risk, there still may be little need to undergo aggressive balloon therapy or surgery. Why have a test that doesn't give you useful information and may lead you to have unnecessary follow-up procedures? Some consumers end up undergoing heart catheterization, despite the fact that they've never had a symptom in their life. Doctors then find a few minor blockages on the angiogram and, in the worst-case scenario, end up sending them for bypass surgery when it's just not indicated.

"It's a revenue generator," says Dr. Steven Nissen, "and those of us who are involved in the politics of medicine, leadership, and organizations like the American Heart Association and the American College of Cardiology are appalled. It's not that calcium scoring can't be used well by sophisticated people. It's that crooks are using it to get people into the cath lab unnecessarily. It's just an outrage that this goes on. Simply put, an overly aggressive cardiologist or surgeon might see some minor blockages and perform angioplasty or bypass for the wrong reasons." Dr. Jeffrey Borer says, simply, that there is no basis for moving from a calcium scan to catheterization in an asymptomatic patient.

The biggest problem in people in their forties is that plaques may not be hard and calcified. In fact, they are likely to be soft plaques, which are most susceptible to fracture and actually lead to heart attacks. The soft plaques aren't calcified and so don't show up at all on the test. Dr. Borer adds, "Ultimately, the atherosclerotic coronary lesions generally will calcify over time, but in young people there hasn't been time for calcification. The forty-year-old with a normal CT may have a fatal MI tomorrow because the plaque that ruptures is a soft plaque that has no calcium." Ironically, the calcified lesion can also be a more stable one, which is less likely to rupture than the newer, small ones.

To be fair, let's look at the proponents' arguments. The biggest and most interesting argument for the scan goes like this. Some heart attacks occur in patients who have only a 40 percent blockage of a coronary artery. That is, even though there is little blockage to blood flow before the heart attack and the patient has no symptoms, the plaque develops a soft spot, which cracks and may cause a heart attack. Therefore, why not find the problem, even though you have no symptoms, and be much more aggressive? We know that medication can help smooth out blockages and stabilize that soft spot. We also know that the progressive closure of the blood vessels may be slowed or even stopped.

So there you have it. This is one of the most intensive debates in modern cardiology. Be prepared for an earful when you bring this up with your doctor. You're unlikely to get a cardiac CT scan if you have no risks or family history. If you do have risk factors, your doctor may argue that he or she is already being aggressive without the scan. It's a good argument. If you're doing everything you can in the most aggressive manner, there's no need for the test. But if you and your doctor need more convincing, the calcium scan could be just the ammunition you're looking for.

A new article in *Circulation* shows that of patients with no symptoms of heart disease who took the test, those with the highest scores were 2.3 times more likely than those with low scores to suffer a fatal heart attack and 10.2 times more likely to need angioplasty or bypass surgery. The most important deciding factor, though, is that calcium scans were a better predictor of risk than conventional risk factors such as cholesterol or blood pressure.

Dr. Matthew Budoff of UCLA, one of the authors of the largest study of EBT scan, says, "I can promise you that the AHA guidelines will be very strong in recommending this test for 'intermediate risk.' Furthermore, the National Cholesterol Education Panel recommends that persons with high calcium scores have more aggressive management of their lipids. The new studies are very strong and very large, reinforcing the idea that calcium buildup in the arteries imparts over tenfold risk of cardiac events."

SHOULD YOU HAVE AN EBT?

The test does have its place as part of your physician's overall game plan. The study of EBT scan found it effective in helping doctors predict heart attacks among patients at intermediate risk. This is the population where there is the biggest problem because there are no symptoms present and the risk isn't classified as high. So we do know that the calcium score correlates fairly well with the overall extent of arterial plaques. This study presented the most compelling data that EBT can predict coronary events with coronary calcium—95 percent of those who had a heart attack had high calcium scores.

As with all tests, you have to ask yourself what you would do with the results. If you are young with no symptoms and only mild risk factors, cardiologists do not advise the test. A high score could lead to two unfavorable outcomes. First, you may end up having surgery or balloon therapy that you do not need. Or you may end up a psychological cardiac cripple, falsely believing that you have serious heart disease.

On the other hand, Dr. Roger Blumenthal counsels that if you are at high risk and have a family history of heart attack, a positive result could lead doctors to be much more aggressive with medical therapy, and this is a real plus. Dr. Blumenthal adds that a stress test and aggressive lifestyle changes plus medication are indicated with a higher score—you should not go directly to the cath lab. A high calcium score also triggers doctors to strongly consider aspirin therapy.

HOW THE TEST IS DONE

It is very simple. You lie down and hold your breath for twenty seconds. There is a small amount of radiation.

WHAT THE TEST RESULTS MEAN

- 400+: Very high, severe plaque burden
- 100–400: High, moderate plaque burden

- 1–100: Mild to moderate (depending on age)
- 0: Clean coronaries, no plaque buildup

THE BOTTOM LINE

If you are at low risk. You don't need EBT, since it's unlikely to uncover disease, say top academics. Studies are ongoing to see if that's true.

If you are at high risk. You should have risk factors treated aggressively no matter what. If you have symptoms, the EBT is redundant since a more precise test should be used to find exactly where the blockages are.

If you are at moderate risk. EBT seems to be most useful in people for whom risk is uncertain and/or are at intermediate risk. EBT may help guide therapeutic or even further diagnostic options.

If you are older. Dr. Steven Nissen counsels, "No one in his or her eighties should ever have a calcium scan. It's absolutely insane because everyone at that age has calcium in the coronaries. Getting these calcium scores in the elderly adds nothing to what we already know." Dr. Scott Grundy, director of the Center for Human Nutrition at the University of Texas Southwestern Medical Center, counters that the test is worth considering in older patients to see if they have a higher amount of calcium compared to the average for their age. Dr. Roger Blumenthal adds that calcium scores add significant independent data to the standard risk factors. Older patients with high calcium should undergo aggressive preventive therapy including the use of statins. My mother's coronaries were white with calcium, but for years her doctors never gave her statins.

If you have chest pain. Consumers Union medical consultants say that EBT should almost never be used to assess chest pain (angina), since it supplies general information about the coronary arteries but none about function or circulation. Dr. Matthew Budoff does make the case that atypical chest pain is one of the more common reasons to order the test.

Summary. The American Heart Association Scientific Committee states that EBT has the greatest potential for further determination of risk particularly in elderly asymptomatic patients and others at intermediate risk.

Still undecided? Here are some more specific pros and cons of the EBT:

PROS

- Calcium shows disease in your coronary arteries and serves as a tiebreaker to determine how aggressively to treat.
- Largest-ever study of EBT scan helps doctors predict heart attacks among patients at intermediate risk.
- Beneficial for "men above the age of forty and women above the age of fifty with at least one traditional risk factor," says Dr. George T. Kondos, lead investigator of the EBT study.
- The test does more than simply identify a risk factor; it can measure the amount of disease by measuring the buildup of calcium in the arteries.
- If you have a zero calcium score, there is only a one in a thousand chance of a heart attack in the next year. That's a pretty good guarantee you have a clean bill of health. The rare exception is the person who smokes, since smoking can cause problems by constricting blood vessels, making blood more likely to clot.

CONS

- Expensive.
- Potential addition of radiation (though the amount of radiation is very small, less than dental x rays).
- Does not supply information about function or circulation in the arteries.
- Can be obtained without a physician's advice or prescription.
- Does not identify calcium in smaller vessels.

In the end, Dr. Diane Bild of the NHLBI argues that if you took those same people who have high calcium scores and instead measured their traditional risk factors—cholesterol, blood pressure, diabetes, smoking, etc.—you might learn the same thing about their risk for having a heart attack. Others argue that calcium is an additional risk factor that can point out trouble when traditional risk factors fail.

ECHOCARDIOGRAM

This is a simple, cheap, and effective method for looking at your heart's structure and function. An echo can't look at your coronary arteries, but it can see if your heart muscle is contracting in a safe and vigorous fashion, and it can pinpoint troubles such as damaged heart valves. The echo works like a ship's sonar. Where a ship sends sound waves to bounce off enemy submarines, a cardiac echo bounces sound waves off the heart's four chambers and four valves.

Your doctor may have you exercise first, then employ the echo while your heart is still beating vigorously to look for abnormal or weak contractions or damaged muscle as a result of a prior heart attack or impaired valve function. He or she may thread an echo down your esophagus to get a more detailed view of the heart, unencumbered by other structures in your chest.

"Echocardiography has opened a window to the heart that is truly marvelous, because you see the heart in real time, and therefore you get a true comprehensive evaluation of someone's heart," says Dr. Miguel A. Quiñones, director of the Baylor Heart Clinic at the Baylor College of Medicine in Waco. New evidence shows that ultrasound can also be used to screen for aneurysms, which may occur in the aorta, your heart's main blood vessel. The ultrasound can find them early enough to save your life.

EJECTION FRACTION

One of the best indicators of the need for aggressive management of heart disease is a measurable decrease in heart function at rest. This can easily be determined with the echocardiogram. Your heart should pump out more than half its contents with each beat. In severe heart disease, it may pump out only 15 percent. By the time you reach 5 percent, if you're still alive, you should be on a heart transplant list.

A depressed ejection fraction increases your risk of congestive heart failure and sudden death. It's important for your doctor to know if your fraction is low. He or she can prescribe ACE inhibitors, beta-blockers, spironolactone, digoxin, and even an implantable cardiodefibrillator (pacemaker) (these are described fully in Steps 6 and 7).

My mother's heart disease was diagnosed with an echocardiogram, which is a wonderful test to follow a patient's progress. Unfortunately, her cardiologist stopped ordering the test, allowing her to fall undetected into severe congestive heart failure.

WHO SHOULD HAVE AN ECHO?

This noninvasive test carries no risk. If your doctor suspects heart disease, he or she can order an echo before proceeding to (or instead of) a riskier test. Also, patients with an enlarged left ventricle are at increased risk for suffering a silent heart attack. The echo is an excellent means of making the diagnosis. Dr. Diane Bild says that left ventricular hypertrophy usually develops after you've had hypertension for some time.

INTRAVASCULAR ULTRASOUND (IVUS)

This research tool is revolutionizing cardiology. The device is threaded into your coronary artery where it can see plaques that are not jutting into the bloodstream—the submerged plaques I talked about at the beginning of this book that do not show up on any other tests. What's alarming is that patients can have dozens of these, which can fracture and cause a fatal heart attack. In addition, follow-up IVUS allows your doctor to see the effect of drugs on these plaques in a matter of days.

RADIONUCLIDE-BASED MYOCARDIAL PERFUSION SCINTIGRAPHY

This test detects blood flow through the heart muscle. That's different from an angiogram (page 120–24), where the heart vessels themselves are clearly outlined. This test helps determine if certain regions of the heart are not getting an adequate amount of blood. Doctors can learn if your heart muscle is or is not functioning properly. The test's chief advantages are that it is safe and can predict your level of risk. The best analogy is that of an overhead satellite photo. It may not be able to see a dried-up riverbed, but it will show that the area it supplied is brown from lack of water rather than green with vegetation.

Also, when the most modern techniques are employed, involving a computerized procedure (called single-photon emission computerized tomography, or SPECT) to provide three-dimensional pictures of the heart, the technique is particularly accurate and even can provide measures of heart function that add to the information available from the perfusion or blood flow data.

HOW THE TEST IS DONE

A technician injects tiny amounts of radioactive material such as thallium 201 or another radioisotope into your bloodstream. Red blood cells pick up the dye and distribute it throughout all the heart muscle. Then a special camera detects the material as it passes through your heart, resulting in an image of the heart. Dr. Jeffrey Borer says, "Though I am admittedly biased, having worked in the area of nuclear cardiology for many years, at present I believe this is the most accurate and predictive of the noninvasive tests for coronary artery disease."

STRESS TEST

Every surgeon I interviewed emphasized the huge amount of silent heart disease that results in heart attacks and death. If you're going to find it easily and effectively, this is the test you want to have.

The old stress test was performed with an EKG alone. That provided an overall picture but did not tell your doctor with any precision where the trouble lay. The new standard stress test employed by many top cardiologists uses radioactive tracers, like thallium or technetium-based perfusion agents described in the previous section, to look at the heart and its blood flow more specifically.

Unlike the old EKG stress test, myocardial perfusion scintigraphy shows major structural defects or important blockages. In fact, says Dr. Jeffrey Borer, the radionuclide-based testing is highly predictive. With the traditional stress test performed with an EKG alone, in a totally asymptomatic patient, even if cholesterol is high, 30–40 percent of positive results will be so-called false positives. That is, the EKG shows heart disease even though you don't have heart disease. With a SPECT myocardial perfusion scintigram with associated ejection fraction determination, you would see perfectly normal blood flow pattern and heart function and have a pretty good idea that it is falsely positive. In talking to cardiologists, I have found that there is no set policy on how you should be stress-tested: an EKG tracing and blood pressure monitoring alone, or a myocardial perfusion scintigram, or an echo.

"If I really thought someone might have important coronary disease, I would do a radionuclide study," says Dr. Jeffrey Borer. When would the old-fashioned EKG stress test alone suffice? "If the person is truly asymptomatic, even if several risk factors for coronary artery disease are present, then it would be reasonable to do an exercise electrocardiogram without the isotope. If the test is completely negative, there is a very high likelihood that the person does not have serious disease. This kind of testing commonly is used to screen people in 'high-risk' jobs, like airline pilots who need to be certain they will not be disabled by a heart attack while flying a plane, or referees for the National Football League, who may be age forty to sixty-five and need to run up and down the football field for several hours during a game. Even so, there are situations in which a radionuclide-based test might be most appropriate for an asymptomatic person."

Adds Dr. Andrew Arai of the NHLBI, "The old test of doing

the stress test and monitoring with an EKG is really a poor test in women." He adds that "an imaging test associated with the stress test can help localize the problems in the heart and makes the test more sensitive than relying on the EKG alone."

WHO SHOULD HAVE A STRESS TEST?

Dr. Lawrence Cohn of Brigham and Women's Hospital states that "if you're a vigorous person, if you have a family history, if you have a genetic influence, if you've had bad diets, if you've smoked—these kind of people probably ought to get a specialist's opinion and an exercise screening test. It's a very excellent way to pick out people who don't have symptoms but still have very severe coronary disease and could drop dead."

If any of the descriptions below apply to you, you probably should have a stress test.

- Beginning a program of vigorous exercise
- Family history
- Genetic predisposition
- Poor diet
- Smoker
- Known heart disease
- Previous heart attack
- Multiple risk factors

EXPERT ADVICE

Dr. Lawrence Cohn: "Let's say you're a man, sixty years old, who wants to start running because he's overweight, etc. A guy like that should get an exercise stress test beforehand so he doesn't go out there and, after about a mile, drop dead from bad coronaries. That's just my personal opinion, it's what I tell my patients."

RADIONUCLIDE CINEANGIOGRAM (RNCA)

This test also uses a radioactive chemical to provide pictures of the heart at rest and during exercise. Though it can provide useful diagnostic information in people with suspected coronary artery disease, and highly accurate predictive information in patients with known or suspected coronary disease, it has been largely superceded by SPECT myocardial perfusion scintigraphy, which has greater diagnostic accuracy. Nonetheless, RNCA is still commonly used, and is very useful, for evaluating patients with valvular heart diseases (especially leaking heart valves), cardiomyopathies, or heart failure.

HOW THE TEST IS DONE

A radioactive tracer is injected into one of your veins. When it reaches the heart, pictures are obtained while you are at rest and again during maximal exercise. (The exercise usually is performed while you are lying on a table and involves pedaling a bicycle attached to the table.) Your doctor will be able to see a movie of the beating heart to determine if your heart pumps out enough blood during each stroke. This is the ejection fraction (see page 111) and generally should be over 50 percent. The movie also allows the doctor to determine if all the different regions of the heart are working properly or if a blocked coronary artery is preventing normal function of some area. You'll also be hooked up to an electrocardiogram to determine if the stress of exercise triggers an irregular heart rhythm or a potentially dangerous oxygen deficit to the heart's pumping muscles.

MRI

Magnetic resonance imaging is being studied by the National Institutes of Health and at several other major imaging centers around the country. The key benefit of an MRI is that it can pick up information in one test that otherwise might require two or more. It's part RNCA scan, part perfusion scintigram, part echo, and part angiogram.

HOW THE TEST IS DONE

You lie down inside a powerful magnet that is turned on for a fraction of a second, causing all the electrically charged molecules in your body to tilt slightly for a split second and then return to their original positions when the magnet is turned off. The tilt and return results in the emission of energy, which is collected by a special detector attached to a computer. Many "pictures" are taken, enabling the computer to provide three-dimensional views of your heart (and other body structures) from this information.

Here's what the MRI can find:

- Like a myocardial perfusion scintigram, the MRI can look at blood supply to heart muscle, detecting those areas where there is little or none.
- Like an echocardiogram or RNCA, the MRI looks at heart function.
- Like a specialized radionuclide scan, the MRI can look at areas of heart attack or damaged heart muscle with a contrast agent called gadolinium.
- Like an angiogram, the MRI can look at the coronary arteries themselves. New studies are beginning to detect the blockages of the coronary arteries. In a head-to-head con-

test, the CT still edges out the MRI for blockages at this time.

Dr. Andrew Arai advises, "The MRI makes the most sense when there is the greatest likelihood of serious heart disease. So if the doctors are thinking that they might need two or more tests to figure out what's wrong with the heart, the MRI can do almost all aspects of what we look for in noninvasive cardiac imaging. It really makes a whole lot of sense."

LOOKING FOR DAMAGE

The MRI makes a huge amount of sense in sorting out whether you have had a heart attack and whether you may benefit from a procedure like angioplasty or bypass surgery. You shouldn't subject yourself to the risk of bypass surgery if, for example, areas of your heart look as if they are permanently damaged. The MRI appears to be the best test for figuring out what portions of the heart are permanently damaged and not likely to improve with that kind of treatment.

EMERGENCY EVALUATION

Another important use of MRI may be in the emergency room. Dr. Andrew Arai reports, "We've looked at using MRI to evaluate patients with chest pain in the emergency room. The test, because it gives such high-quality images, looks like it's going to be one of the best tests, although it's still in the validation stages for ER work.

"It's a very interesting idea because here we're using a state-of-the-art imaging tool and finding things in patients that the standard tests are missing. I think people are amazed by just how much gets missed in the emergency department with chest pain patients with the current EKG tests.

"There are fundamental limitations to the kinds of tests that we run. An EKG is a great tool when it works, when it gives the answer, but it's just not sensitive enough, it misses a fair number of things. And the blood tests are fantastic for picking up a heart attack, but they miss what we call an impending heart attack, or unstable angina."

SCREENING

Dr. Diane Bild warns that the MRI is not ready for use as a screening test. "The MRI is a very sophisticated test and is very expensive. I can't imagine that it would be considered in the realm of some type of a screening test in the near future. What you get from the MRI is a very detailed anatomical description of the heart, you get a beautiful picture of its structure, and you get information about its function. But it's actually not that good at picking up coronary artery disease in asymptomatic people.

"Some new MRI angiographies, called MRA techniques, are being developed. Those may at some point be useful off the street. One thing that's good about MRI is that it's totally noninvasive—that is, if you don't get a contrast injection with it—and there is no radiation exposure. Still it's unlikely to be used as a general screening test in the near future."

ELECTROPHYSIOLOGY STUDY (EPS)

There are three kinds of damage to your heart. First, the heart muscle may be damaged by a heart attack or by other processes, like infection, trauma, or genetic abnormalities, that are expressed only as you grow older. Second, the heart's valves may be damaged by a severe heart attack, congenital defect, or other disease process. Third, your heart's electrical system may be damaged, either by one of the processes involved in damaging the heart muscle or valves, or by an abnormality affecting the electrical system alone. This damage to the electrical system can be instantly fatal.

You or your doctor may have noticed irregular heart rhythms. Your doctor may take several steps. A twenty-four-hour recording on a Holter monitor will reveal irregularities at any time of day or night. An EKG stress test may also provoke abnormalities in parts of the electrical system starved for oxygen. But in certain situations, the best way to determine the precise nature of the problem is with a highly specialized test performed in a catheterization laboratory. This electrophysiology study (or EPS) stresses your heart's electrical system to elicit dangerous irregularities of heart rhythm such as ventricular tachycardia.

The EPS is not appropriate for routine applications; there the twenty-four-hour EKG is still the test of choice. If you notice irregular heartbeat, be sure to have your doctor detect what kind they are. Many are perfectly benign, but others can kill you. New implantable defibrillators are among the treatments for dangerous arrhythmias.

ANGIOGRAM:
THE GOLD STANDARD

What if your screening tests spell trouble? If your doctor suspects that you have serious heart disease after a stress test with or without radioisotope, there is only one test that indicates with certainty exactly what's going on in your coronary arteries: an angiogram. It is the only test with enough precision to guide doctors in undertaking balloon therapy or bypass surgery.

Traditionally the catheterization was a dangerous invasive procedure that took several hours. You came in the day before, then you stayed in the hospital another day or two after the test. Unless you were sick enough to require surgery, you didn't undergo catheterization. Nowadays, you come in as an outpatient; have the catheterization, which takes 30 to 40 minutes at most; then go home. The ease and safety, however, do lure many more patients to have the test, some of whom should avoid it.

When doctors do studies to determine if coronary artery disease has been reversed, they also rely on the angiogram. For superprecision, researchers can use a tiny ultrasound tip on a catheter placed in the coronary artery to measure the exact thickness of a blockage. Routine angiograms can miss many life-threatening blockages that are not big enough to appear dangerous. (Only the intravascular ultrasound shows multiple life-threatening blockages coursing through an entire coronary artery that are too small to appear as significant blockages on the angiogram. Unfortunately, the intravascular ultrasound is still just a research tool.)

HOW THE TEST IS DONE

A long, thin, hollow-tipped tube called a catheter is hooked up to a pressure recorder and a source of contrast medium that usually contains iodine. (There are several non-iodine-containing contrast media available for people allergic to iodine.) That contrast medium is a liquid that X-rays cannot pass through. The cardiologist then uses a needle to make a small hole in an artery in your leg or arm and threads the catheter into progressively larger arteries until it reaches the aortic valve (the

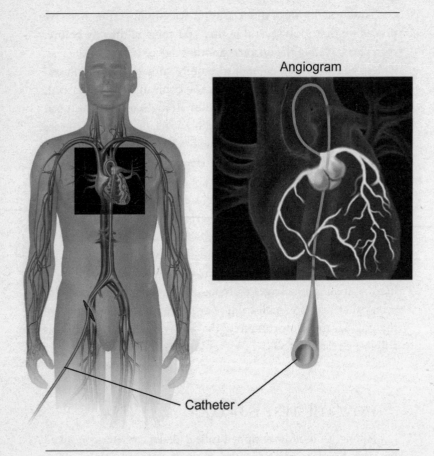

Angiogram

Catheter

valve that leads out of the heart's main pumping chamber, the left ventricle, into the aorta). The doctor manipulates the catheter so that the tip is inserted into the origin of each of the two coronary arteries. Once inside, the first objective is to be certain that the pressure in the coronary artery is the same as in the aorta. If the pressure is low or drops after the doctor engages, that means blood isn't flowing the way it should to maintain the arterial pressure.

The cardiologist then injects the contrast medium into your arteries. When an X-ray tries to pierce through your body, the contrast medium stops it dead in its tracks, and the picture shows up as white where the contrast is. Your doctor can see the complete coronary artery tree. To go back to the satellite analogy, it is like an overhead photo of a river and all its tributaries. If one tributary were blocked, it would show up on the photo. So where that column of contrast medium is partially or totally obstructed, there is a blockage shown on the angiogram.

"That's how you define where the blockages are in the coronary arteries, how severe they are, whether the remainder of the artery is in a condition that could make it technically suitable for a bypass grafting procedure, and whether the blockage is of sufficient size and shape so that it could be amenable to an angioplasty," says Dr. Jeffrey Borer. "All those things can be judged from the picture you've just taken. It's the only test that can give you these answers. Notice I didn't say whether you 'should' do bypass or angioplasty, I said whether you 'could' perform one of these procedures. Whether or not you *should* do the procedure requires evaluation of clinical information (the result of a history and physical examination), often integrated with the results of noninvasive testing."

That's a key point. The angiogram shows surgeons and cardiologists the technical feasibility of treating your disease with balloon therapy or surgery and outlines the approaches they could use and the difficulty they could expect to encounter. With multiple injections, the camera can be moved into different positions for different views of the heart. This is important because the coronary arteries are not straight tubes headed in one direction. They are irregularly shaped vessels that turn in many different directions. If you don't take multiple pictures from multiple angles, you may miss an obstruction.

It's always important clinically to know the status of the heart's function and, most important, of the main pumping chamber (left ventricle). For that reason, a motion picture of the left ventricle is made, as is a record of the left ventricular pressure.

MAJOR RISKS

The most obvious risk is that when you put a tube into a blood vessel or into the heart, you could puncture either. That's uncommon, because the doctors who do these procedures are very well trained and highly skilled. Still, it does happen.

Infection can be introduced into the blood vessels when the catheter passes through the skin if the skin hasn't been cleaned off properly. Bacteria can also make their way into the bloodstream if they are in the air in the catheterization suite. This is also very uncommon.

Blood clots can form inside the catheter, or if the catheter scrapes along the side of the heart or along the side of a vessel in a certain way, causing a small injury, a blood clot may form at the sight of the injury. The blood thinner heparin may help prevent these clots from forming once the catheter is in place.

A heart attack was a major and common complication of an angiogram twenty years ago. Though much less common today, the catheter may injure the lining of the artery or block the artery, causing a heart attack. This is why you don't want to have an angiogram for frivolous reasons. It should be done as a planning test for an indicated procedure.

The contrast medium itself can occlude the blood flow through the arteries sufficiently long in a sufficiently ill person to cause a heart attack or an irregular heart rhythm. Some arrhythmias, such as ventricular tachycardia, can be lethal. That's why defibrillators are placed in the catheterization suite on standby.

There can be allergic reactions to the dye, which contains iodine. Be sure to tell your doctor if you are allergic to iodine or seafood. Doctors can use a nonionic medium or pretreat you with steroids.

SHOULD YOU HAVE AN ANGIOGRAM?

If your doctor is seriously considering a bypass grafting procedure or an angioplasty, you must first have an angiogram. However, Dr. Jeffrey Borer advises, "Don't delay your decision about whether to do a procedure until after the angiogram. I don't! I use other tests to determine prognosis and use the catheterization basically as a road map for treatment." Like Dr. Borer, I suggest that you gather as much information as possible from the tests you've read about in this chapter and the last before committing to an angiogram unless your doctor feels that your life is in imminent danger.

Dr. Borer warns that there is a very low threshold for ordering an angiogram, "in part because we've trained so many interventional cardiologists, who need to do a certain number of cases each year to stay current and who truly believe that the angiogram is the best procedure as a basis for decisions. Remember, when you have a hammer, there is a tendency for everything you see to look like a nail. So there's a big incentive to go ahead and do these procedures. And I think that's of real concern."

Dr. Thomas Graboys recounts, "Every week I see second-opinion patients who are feeling fine, but they went and had an exercise test. The exercise test was positive, and they were told, 'You've got some narrowing, some blockages.' And as soon as they hear that, they say, 'Okay, fix them.' Well, they have the cath, which shows 80 to 90 percent circulation, so we're not looking at life-threatening anatomies. Still, they go in and have a stent placed. Patients had minimal symptoms before, now they have a stent in, and psychologically they go from being terrified to being less than terrified and thankful that the doc saved their lives by opening up this narrowed vessel. It's a battlefield out there and there are stray bullets, people get hit by friendly fire—that's part of a reality. How many caths are done because the interventional cardiologist at that particular hospital hasn't done enough cases this month or this year?"

That's why you want to be certain that the angiogram is appropriate. Here, however, is how it gets even more tricky. Surgeons like Harvard's Lawrence Cohn and Cornell's Wayne Isom have seen countless angiograms showing significant, even potentially lethal blockage in people who didn't appear to be candidates for surgery. If your tests are equivocal and you're not certain about getting an angiogram, this is the time to see an expert cardiologist at a top center.

ARRHYTHMIAS

These are irregularities of the heartbeat. Most are benign and don't require treatment, but they still need to be tested to be sure. You may be asked to wear a Holter monitor for a twenty-four-hour period to see if you have irregular heart rhythms during your activities of daily living. If the irregularity requires treatment but is straightforward, your doctor may elect to treat you on the basis of this test alone. If you have a more dangerous or complicated problem, you'll be sent to a catheterization laboratory where doctors will directly stress your heart's electrical system to explore its vulnerabilities.

On the basis of these studies, your doctor can consider correcting the disorder with drugs, surgery, electric shock, or even an implantable defibrillator and pacemaker. The key here is proper diagnosis and treatment by an expert in arrhythmias at a major academic center.

The tests in this chapter are what the missing half never get to. These tests would give them the definitive diagnosis necessary to know what disease they have and beat it before it beats them.

The bottom line is that the best test is the one that shows your entire coronary artery tree in great detail. Right now, only angiography, with all its risks, allows doctors to do that. Doctors are looking at a totally noninvasive scan, which yields a full map of the coronary arteries during exercise. This way doctors see every last nook and cranny and can detect important disease quickly and easily.

STEP SIX: TAKE LIFESAVING MEDICATIONS

Fatal Flaw

"Your father's in the hospital, he's had a heart attack." I froze, then my heart started to race. What could I do? The man I loved most in the world could die at any moment. I finally reached the doctor treating him at the hospital by phone. Her voice was very cheery, but I was not reassured. I got the impression that this was not a big deal to her. What was wrong? He had a bout of acute congestive heart failure. In a word, he was drowning from fluid that was filling his lungs. Soon she started him on digitalis and furosemide (Lasix), among the standard therapies for heart failure. There were also recent laboratory tests indicating a heart attack.

I called a top expert in heart failure at Brigham and Women's Hospital. What could be done? She was very comforting. There was lots: A series of new developments dramatically increased the quality and duration of life for heart failure patients; there were medications that made the heart work better, others that prevented fatal disturbances of the heart rhythm. Relieved and grateful, I called my father's cardiologist. He took a mild interest but brushed aside my suggestions, saying I should clear them with his primary care doctor at the time in a suburban Boston hospital. Without the backing of his primary doctor, I knew it was a tough sell.

I reviewed the plan of the heart failure expert at Brigham and Women's hospital and suggested that my father see her. His cardiologist listened intently and said he'd bring it up with my father and his primary care provider. Despite my pleas, he never saw the heart failure expert. A key part of the strategy would have been to give him medications that could prevent sudden cardiac death—precisely what eventually killed him.

My father saw top Harvard-educated doctors and was a Harvard Medical School graduate himself. Yet even he had difficulty getting the right medications at the best institutions in the country. This was several years before he died. He already took a handful of medications but lacked those that could help prevent sudden death or extend his life.

I can't emphasize this last point strongly enough. Most patients are happy taking the nuts-and-bolts medications that give them symptomatic relief. Far too few have the foresight to take the extra medications whose sole effect is increasing life expectancy.

Cardiology is a highly specialized part of internal medicine, and these specialists have specialties. As Dr. Jeffrey Borer articulates, the very explosion of knowledge about heart disease has

Conventional wisdom: *I'm on the right meds.*
The real deal: *Don't count on it. The vast majority of patients are not taking the right doses of the right drugs. At least half of those and as many as 90 percent who should be on medications are not taking any at all. Hundreds of thousands pay the ultimate price.*

created a knowledge gap. Your doctor may be terrific at treating your heart's electrical system but miss treating a weakened heart. You could have a fabulously skilled cardiologist when it comes to balloon therapy but he or she misses reducing your cholesterol enough to avoid the next major blockage. How can you be certain you're getting a comprehensive plan for heart health?

This chapter is designed to make you a good consumer: to know the kinds of drugs you should be asking your doctor about and the kinds of results you should expect. Medications don't have the same allure as the high-tech wizardry of balloon therapy, but they work miracles by protecting millions from having a fatal heart attack.

As you'll see, we're entering a new era when heart disease can be slowed, stopped, and even reversed with the proper application of medication and lifestyle. There is a three-way race on among surgery, balloon therapy, and medications. Medications, long a dull backwater, are now surging to the front of the pack with the ability to dramatically alter the course of your disease, drying up the toxic cholesterol cores of the blockages found in your arteries and toughening the fibrous capsule to prevent a heart attack. This is incredibly important, since balloon therapy picks off just one, two, or three blockages at a time whereas intravascular ultrasound may show dozens of important and life-threatening plaques lining your coronary arteries.

The future of medications, says Dr. Steven Nissen, is that of cocktail therapy: the use of many different medications to provide a spectacular result. Many cancers are cured by cocktail therapy, and that appears to be the future of heart disease as well.

When taking medications, as often as possible look for drugs that have a secondary benefit. For instance, beta-blockers have a primary benefit of preventing chest pain but also a secondary benefit, in patients who have had a heart attack, of preventing additional heart attacks and death. It's not enough to treat today's symptoms; you want to treat for long-term success.

This chapter contains a lot of technical details. Here's how to use it. As an example, say you are already taking a statin but discover that adding niacin could dramatically affect your overall cholesterol screen. Your concern is lowering your cholesterol, so you want details about the actual medications for this condition and to see whether it makes sense to speak with your doctor about adding drugs to your regimen. In this way the chapter serves both as a guideline and a reference section. The key is building awareness of drugs that may benefit you.

The chapter is divided as follows so you can home in on the actual clinical problems you have:

- Drugs That Prevent Blood Clots
- Drugs That Lower Cholesterol
- Drugs That Lower High Blood Pressure
- Drugs That Treat Coronary Artery Disease
- Drugs That Treat Congestive Heart Failure
- Supplements

The first two sections are for anyone with risk factors for heart disease. The sections on blood pressure, coronary artery disease, and congestive heart failure provide detailed information for patients diagnosed with those actual conditions.

KNOW THE RIGHT MEDICATIONS AND HOW TO USE THEM

How do you know which medications really work? Target treatment goals and expanding drug treatment guidelines are based on the results of elaborate, expensive, and well-designed studies called clinical trials. Expert clinical judgment further refines their use. Where possible, this chapter uses the latest, biggest, and best clinical trials along with the knowledge of top academic experts.

CUSTOMIZED DRUGS

There is no one-size-fits-all plan for treating heart disease. Each patient has different genetics and risk factors, and that means unique prescriptions for medications. Take high blood pressure. There are a boatload of drugs that can reduce your blood pressure. However, some tend to cause hard-to-tolerate side effects while others have complementary actions that help reduce your other risks of heart disease. Other drugs are too expensive. This chapter takes a highly tactical approach, looking first at medications that prevent a heart attack, then at medications that treat heart disease and heart failure.

The goal of this chapter is not to replace the many excellent books on medications currently available in bookstores—and certainly not to replace your doctor—but to lay out the rationale for drug use and to give you guidelines to make you aware of medications that may help you most. If you know which drugs could benefit you most, you're ahead of 90 percent of patients.

COMPLIANCE

The most important problem in modern pharmacology is that of patient compliance. Some patients think that if one pill is good, two pills are better; others decide they don't feel so bad, and they cut their dosage in half. Even patients who begin following the prescribed treatment stop taking their drugs on their own, not taking them long enough to save their lives.

If you take home only one point from this chapter, it is to continue taking your medications as they are prescribed for as long as they are prescribed. Once the majority of patients are on the right drug (or drugs), they usually do not take enough of it long enough to make a difference. A relative of mine with high cholesterol believed that by cutting his dose of a statin, he was being judicious. As a diabetic, he sharply increased his risk. My mother wants to stop taking medications almost as soon as she starts taking them. "That's our biggest problem," says Dr. James McKenney of the Department of Pharmacy at Virginia Commonwealth University. "Patients drop out of therapy and they don't get the benefits. The benefits, in terms of fewer heart attacks and strokes, don't come till at least six months out or more."

Despite the almost miraculous qualities of the cholesterol-lowering drugs called statins, as many as 50 percent of patients stop taking them after just one year. Part of this is due to a fear of side effects. "It seems that it has a lot to do with your own personal sense of risk and personal sense of whether it's a good or bad thing to take a little pill every morning," says Dr. Dennis Sprecher.

DRUGS THAT PREVENT BLOOD CLOTS

The last event leading to a heart attack is the formation of a blood clot that blocks off the final trickle of blood flow through a coronary artery, starving the heart of nutrients and killing the heart's muscle. Here are the drugs that can prevent those blood clots from forming in your heart's arteries.

ASPIRIN

Cheap, widely available, and underestimated, this miracle drug of yesteryear is still the miracle drug of today, though largely overlooked as an important therapeutic agent in the battle against heart disease. The highest quality of clinical trials have proved that aspirin can save lives in a variety of situations from basic prevention to the emergency treatment of a heart attack. It's old and low-tech, but aspirin can lower your risk of heart attack nearly as much as lowering your cholesterol can. Aspirin reduces the risk of heart disease by an astonishing 28 percent.

These are the primary indications for aspirin:

Heart attack. Aspirin is usually given to patients who arrive in the emergency department with a suspected heart attack. Aspirin may decrease the size of a blood clot during a heart attack by preventing the clumping of platelets, the basic building blocks of a blood clot.

After bypass surgery and balloon therapy. Patients treated with aspirin have fewer early closures of the newly grafted or opened blood vessels in their hearts.

Post–heart attack. Aspirin decreases the risk of heart attack in those who have already had one.

Primary prevention. If you don't have heart disease and are at low risk, the use of preventive aspirin is controversial. The conventional wisdom is that everyone over fifty might just as well pop an aspirin a day. As you'll see, the choice should be made more carefully. There are excellent data about the efficacy of aspirin during an acute MI in patients who have suffered a previous heart attack, and even among patients with angina without prior MI. However, data about primary prevention—that is, in people without known heart disease—while highly suggestive, are not conclusive given the risks. The FDA Cardiorenal Advisory Committee voted against extending the aspirin label to indicate its use for "primary prevention" of heart attacks in "moderate-risk" patients (those with high cholesterol, high blood pressure, and other risk factors but without clinically evident disease).

RISKS

Aspirin is not risk free. It can increase the risk of hemorrhagic strokes or major gastrointestinal bleeding. To put that into perspective, aspirin would prevent fourteen heart attacks over a five-year period in a thousand high-risk patients, but one would suffer a stroke and three would suffer gastrointestinal bleeding. In lower-risk patients, over the same five-year period, three heart attacks would be prevented but one person would suffer a stroke and five would experience major gastrointestinal bleeding.

Bottom line, consider your net benefit. If you're at high risk, there's lots of benefit. If you're at low risk, there's more risk than benefit. How do you calculate that risk? The Framingham score is still the best (see "What Is Your Risk?" on pages 92–102). A 5 percent risk over ten years is considered high and a 1 percent risk is considered low.

The risk from aspirin is monumentally higher than that from statins. You should seriously consider aspirin as part of your plan to prevent a heart attack, as long as you calculate this risk carefully. The U.S. Preventive Services Task Force strongly recommends that clinicians discuss the use of aspirin to prevent coronary heart disease with patients who are at increased risk. Aspirin helps prevent the predominant kind of stroke, that caused by a blood clot, but it may cause the less common bleeding stroke. While there is potential therapy for a stroke caused by a clot, little that can be done to actively treat a stroke caused by bleeding.

Bleeding strokes. As many as two patients per 1,000 individuals given aspirin for five years suffer a bleeding or hemorrhagic stroke. Unfortunately, there is no way to predict the risk of a stroke based on preexisting heart disease, dosage of aspirin, or duration of treatment. However, age seems to be a factor: older patients face a greater risk from aspirin therapy.

Gastrointestinal bleeding. This risk also increases with age, regardless of the dosage of aspirin. The rate of major gastrointestinal bleeding episodes is 2 to 4 per 1,000 middle-aged individuals over five years. The use of enteric-coated or buffered preparations does not appear to reduce risk. Taking other nonsteroidal anti-inflammatory agents such as ibuprofen or anticoagulants increases the risk. Ulcer medications such as Prilosec or Zantac may lower the risk of taking aspirin.

Aspirin is cheap and taking it seems to be a real no-brainer. However, take a close look at your personal risk-benefit profile before you decide to pop one.

Age. In at least one trial, aspirin reduced the risk of heart attack as much as or even more than for patients seventy to eighty-four as those fifty to sixty-nine.

Sex. The effect of aspirin on men vs. women is not yet clear. The Women's Health Initiative (WHI) study did not show a significant preventive effect for women. Other large trials of aspirin for primary prevention generally didn't study women. The Women's Health Study, testing low-dose aspirin in 40,000 patients, is expected to clarify the risks and benefits.

Diabetes. Several trials show that patients with diabetes benefit as much as and potentially a great deal more than patients without diabetes.

High blood pressure. Aspirin does not work as well in patients with high blood pressure. The poorer the control of your blood pressure, the less effective aspirin appears to be. Although they do not technically go hand in hand, good blood pressure control does allow aspirin to work better. This is another reason to control your blood pressure to get the maximum preventive effect.

HOW ASPIRIN WORKS

Aspirin works in two key ways. It prevents blood clots by making platelets less sticky. Platelets, as you've seen, are an essential building block of blood clots, which can block coronary arteries and cause a heart attack.

Aspirin also decreases general inflammation. Inflammation of blood vessels is a newly recognized, important factor in heart disease. Proponents believe that aspirin may help reduce this inflammation. Dr. Steven Nissen, however, is not yet persuaded and calls this controversial.

DOSE

A baby aspirin (81 mg) can be just as effective at blocking platelet clumping as a large-dose pill. Platelets aggregating is the core of a blood clot. Aspirin inhibits the key platelet aggregation factor thromboxane at very low dose. This lower dose might also put you at lower risk for gastrointestinal bleeding and hemorrhagic stroke. This is a clear case of less is more. Since you're getting the basic inhibiting effect at such a low dose, there's rarely a reason to go higher. No evidence has been found to support an aspirin dose greater than 325 mg, and dosages as low as 75 mg have been found to be equally effective. Dr. James Atkins adds, "If you're looking for the antiplatelet effect of aspirin, that remains at high level for forty-eight hours after a single dose. So you can take a baby aspirin every other day and get the antiplatelet effect. Be aware, however, that most major clinical trials did use the larger-dose 325-mg tablet."

BOTTOM LINE

The American Heart Association recommends aspirin for patients with a higher risk of coronary artery disease, especially those whose ten-year risk is 10 percent or higher. If you are at low risk, your risk of complications from aspirin outweighs any benefit you might receive. Instead, consider statins.

OTHER DRUGS THAT AFFECT BLOOD CLOTTING

CLOPIDOGREL (PLAVIX)

This is another antiplatelet agent. Patients who are resistant to or cannot tolerate aspirin should strongly consider clopidogrel if they are at substantial risk for heart disease. Can aspirin be taken with clopidogrel? Yes. Patients presenting with a recent acute coronary syndrome, especially after balloon therapy, can benefit.

The long-term use of clopidogrel is limited by the expense. Says Dr. Gary Francis, director of the Coronary Intensive Care Unit at the Cleveland Clinic, "It's a hardship. It costs $75 a month to take it, and for some people that's too much. Some people won't even fill the prescription when the pharmacist tells them that it's going to be expensive. Also, clopidogrel is more likely to cause bleeding than is aspirin, so, again, risk-benefit issues must be considered."

Still, says Dr. Jeffrey Borer, "Clopidogrel is more potent than aspirin in preventing blood clots and therefore people who have had a recent heart attack can benefit from clopidogrel. People who've had unstable angina can benefit from clopidogrel too."

Could clopidogrel be better than aspirin? There are certain situations following acute events where clopidogrel might be preferable, such as after an angioplasty, though the studies to support that aren't the most rigorous.

If clopidogrel is used with aspirin, the CURE (Clopidogrel in Unstable Angina to Prevent Recurrent Events) trial researchers show that higher doses of aspirin do not decrease the risk of heart attacks but do increase the risk of major bleeding episodes. Clopidogrel is seen as a superdrug, despite the risk, especially in sick patients and those undergoing surgical procedures.

DOSE

One 75-mg tablet daily is the only dose that's been studied.

WARFARIN (COUMADIN)

This is a "blood thinner" used to prevent blood clots. Actually, it doesn't really "thin" the blood; it reduces the amount of certain proteins that are central to the clotting process. Warfarin is used in patients with atrial fibrillation or deep vein inflammation (phlebitis), after implantation of artificial heart valves, after some kinds of strokes, or, sometimes, after a heart attack, as well as in certain other settings.

Many patients believe that they do not need to take aspirin if they are taking warfarin. Since aspirin and warfarin have different effects on the blood, there can be an increased benefit to taking both. In one study, patients receiving both aspirin and warfarin had a 29 percent reduced risk, compared to only a 19 percent reduction in those who took warfarin alone. The results, however, were not statistically significant; in other words, it is not possible to say for sure that they weren't just due to chance. Studies are trying to determine if warfarin will help patients with sinus rhythm disturbances or a depressed ejection fraction. If you're taking warfarin for atrial fibrillation, as an example, you could still benefit from aspirin because aspirin works by a different mechanism.

Note: Warfarin (Coumadin) interacts with more than 100 other medications, and with some herbal supplements. Be sure your doctor knows *everything* else you are taking, so that he or she can adjust dosages.

DRUGS THAT LOWER CHOLESTEROL

STATINS

These are the most powerful and important drugs currently available for those who have blockages in their coronary arteries. The ability of statins to lower levels of bad LDL is unprecedented. Their most powerful outcome is the proven ability to reduce your chance of having a heart attack or stroke, or requiring bypass surgery or balloon therapy. They are easy to take, are well accepted by patients, and have few interactions with other drugs or side effects. Studies have reported 20 to 60 percent lower LDL cholesterol levels in patients on statins. Some statins also reduce triglyceride levels and produce a modest increase in good cholesterol levels.

Why do statins work better than any other drugs? They inhibit the key enzyme that controls the rate of cholesterol production in the liver. Statins also increase the liver's ability to remove the LDL cholesterol already in the blood. Since most of your cholesterol is made by your body, rather than coming from what you eat, this is the most important method of achieving substantial reductions in blood cholesterol. So convinced are the experts of its benefits that they have issued new guidelines increasing the numbers of Americans targeted for cholesterol-lowering drugs from 13 million to 36 million.

When these cholesterol-lowering statins first came out, I did a television segment for CBS's *This Morning,* featuring a middle-aged man. For the first time in years, he finally achieved a normal cholesterol reading. He had tried every medication and diet. I asked him what he liked best about taking this new class of drugs. He looked at me mischievously and said, "Oh, let me see, burgers, fries, shakes, Boston cream pie." He kidded about opening a line of steak houses where he'd serve filet mignon as an entrée and statins for dessert! His doctor was miffed, because he had given the patient strict instructions about diet and exercise. Still, the patient's record low cholesterol level had him very excited.

Don't think that if you pop a statin along with a bacon cheeseburger you cancel out the effects of the beef. The saturated fats found in red meats increase your chance of MI, even if you are on statins. That's because saturated fats can harm the key endothelial cells after even a *single meal*. Remember, endothelial cells produce chemicals that allow blood vessels to dilate. Saturated fats damage the production of these chemicals and the endothelial cells. For men, that's even more important, since anything that damages endothelial function hurts erectile function.

THE STATIN REVOLUTION

If you have any risk factors for heart disease, the question is not should you take statins. The question is why would you *not* want to be on them.

Remodeling. The most compelling reason to take statins is that they may help remodel the blockages most of us already have in our coronary arteries. Statins may stabilize plaques by decreasing the LDL cholesterol in the plaque, reshaping the plaque and allowing its exterior coat to become tougher and less susceptible to fracture.

As you learned, this may be the single most important way to prevent a heart attack. If there is one point you take home from this chapter, it's that statins are the new aspirin. Where for years many of us popped an aspirin every day to prevent a heart attack, we should now think of popping a statin in nearly the same cavalier fashion. Why? Statins are *far* safer than aspirin and should be considered your first-line measure to prevent heart disease, even if you have average cholesterol. The FDA is being petitioned to allow statins to be sold over the counter. I believe that statins are safer than aspirin and may play a more important preventive role.

Anti-inflammatory. Statins have profound anti-inflammatory effects. New research shows that heart disease is not a result only of high cholesterol levels but also of inflammation in the lining of coronary arteries, as you learned in the section on inflammation. This means that statins can benefit people who have inflammatory factors even with so-called normal cholesterol levels. Reducing the amount of inflammation in the areas where there is plaque is important because we now know that inflammation is an important contributor to instability of the plaque and the risk of going on to have a heart attack. As a direct measure of inflammation, statins have been shown to lower CRP levels.

Average cholesterol levels. No matter what your cholesterol is, if you have high risk for coronary disease or have coronary disease, your cholesterol could be lower. There is still emerging data in a huge study from the United Kingdom showing that even if your cholesterol is incredibly low, if you lowered it farther, you'd do substantially better over the next several years than if you didn't take statins. That's true not only if you have coronary disease but also if you just have high risk of coronary disease. The CARE trial demonstrated that lowering a mildly elevated cholesterol reduced heart attack by 24 percent in high-risk patients. What's mildly elevated? An LDL of 139 mg/dL.

However, a study published in *The Lancet* in 2002 may revolutionize the way statins are prescribed. The study found remarkable benefits even in high-risk patients with low cholesterol levels. That has led Professor Sir Charles George, medical director of the British Heart Foundation, to coin the slogan, "Treat risk, not cholesterol level."

SIDE EFFECTS

Some patients won't take statins or else they limit their dose for fear of serious side effects. Much of this fear was generated by press reports linking up to 100 deaths from severe destruction of muscle to a drug called Baycol. Baycol has been removed from the market. There is no indication that other statins have anything but the rarest risk of death. The rates of severe myopathy (muscle damage) are equivalently low among all of the approved statins currently on the market.

Statins are remarkably risk-free medications. Nonetheless, you'll want to know about the chief risk factor since it could pose a real threat. Patients commonly complain about nonspecific muscle aches or joint pains. If your blood test is negative for muscle breakdown products, statins are not likely to cause serious long-term problems. The rate of complaints is about 5 percent of those taking the drug. Since 5 percent of patients not taking statins also have the same complaints, the suggestion is that the muscle and joint aches are largely unrelated to the drug.

What doctors worry about most is a rare severe myositis. The symptoms are muscle aches, soreness, or weakness. The giveaway is a lab test showing that levels of the enzyme creatine kinase have risen more than ten times normal. This is the most important indication to stop taking the drug. Failure to discontinue drug therapy can lead to rhabdomyolysis, myoglobinuria, and acute renal necrosis—in lay terms, muscle begins to self-destruct. The debris enters the bloodstream, clogging the kidneys and causing them to fail. This is extremely serious and it's why doctors need to be vigilant, but it is also rare; one death per million prescriptions, according to a detailed analysis by the FDA of their Adverse Event Reporting System.

Dr. Dennis Sprecher points out that a study of statin usage for a sizable number of initially treated people in the 1980s is at the fifteen- to seventeen-year mark in terms of demonstrated safety. Lack of a cancer signal after the twenty-year mark is thought pivotal in defining nondrug-associated cancer risk.

A chemical hepatitis may develop in as many as 10 percent of patients. This is reversible if the drug is stopped.

PREVENTING SIDE EFFECTS

Are you at risk of side effects? This list will help you determine if you are.

- Age: more than 80 years, especially in women
- Small body frame
- Frailty
- Diseases affecting multiple body organs, such as chronic kidney disease or diabetes
- Before and after surgery
- Multiple medications
- Specific medications:
  - amiodarone
  - azole antifungals (itraconazole, ketoconazole)
  - cyclosporine
  - fibrates (gemfibrozil tops the list)
  - HIV protease inhibitors
  - macrolide antibiotics (erythromycin, clarithromycin)
  - nefazodone (antidepressant)
  - nicotinic acid (niacin) (rare)
  - verapamil
- Excessive alcohol consumption

What precautions can your doctor take if this list finds you at greater risk? The best advice is to limit the dose of statins to just that required to reach your therapeutic goal. If you're undergoing surgery, stop taking statins until you have recovered.

MONITORING STATIN USE

As risk-free as statins are for most people, they still require follow-up for specific symptoms or problems.

Headache, indigestion. See your doctor if the symptoms persist. Then follow up six to eight weeks after starting therapy and at each subsequent visit.

Muscle soreness, tenderness, or pain. Your doctor should order a creatine kinase measurement.

Unusual levels of liver enzymes. ALT (alanine transferase) and AST (aspartate transferase) are both levels of liver enzymes. HMG-CoA reductase inhibitors, like some other lipid-lowering therapies, have been associated with biochemical abnormalities of liver function. Your doctor will evaluate your ALT/AST initially, approximately twelve weeks after starting therapy, and then semiannually or more often if indicated.

WHEN TO USE STATINS

After balloon therapy. After you've had stents placed in your coronary arteries, statins are recommended to prevent new disease from occurring. A recent Dutch study published in *JAMA* showed that the incidence of heart attacks was more then 20 percent lower in patients who were given a statin after balloon therapy than in patients who did not receive statins. Dr. George Sopko of the NHLBI says that statins appear to have a double benefit of helping promote artery healing after angioplasty and helping keep arteries clear of new fatty deposits.

After bypass surgery. Bypass surgery by itself does nothing to halt the progression of coronary artery disease. You may get a clean start, but the bypass grafts run the risk of becoming clogged again over the years. That's why surgeons want to aggressively lower your bad cholesterol after surgery. Bypass grafts will last a good deal longer, and that could mean avoiding repeat surgery years down the road.

By way of background, coronary artery bypass surgery uses either saphenous veins taken from the legs, the internal mammary artery from the chest or, less common, the radial artery from the wrist or even the gastroepiploic artery from the abdomen. An NHLBI study published in the *New England Journal of Medicine* observed only saphenous veins bypass. Just like coronary arteries, vein grafts become blocked with accumulations of cholesterol. "This study provides a definitive answer to the question of whether coronary bypass grafts respond to cholesterol lowering similarly to coronary arteries. Furthermore, it is clear from this research that the degree of LDL cholesterol lowering is a critical factor in atherosclerosis progression," Dr. Claude Lenfant said. On the lower dose, 39 percent of patients experienced progression of their atherosclerosis. On the higher dose, only 29 percent of patients showed progression. This gives doctors a clear mandate to aggressively lower LDL cholesterol levels in the 300,000-plus heart disease patients undergoing coronary artery bypass surgery every year in the United States.

Without therapy, about 50 percent of saphenous bypass grafts become blocked ten to twelve years after surgery. Those at highest risk are patients with high cholesterol levels. As a result, these patients may need a repeat bypass or balloon therapy. The target LDL level of the higher-dose group was below 85 mg/dL. For the lower dose-group, the target LDL level was 130 to 140 mg/dL.

Cholestyramine was added to the statin therapy if patients didn't come close enough to their target LDL level. All patients were also encouraged to take a baby aspirin (81 mg) each day.

Diabetes. Statins are also a must for patients with diabetes, who have a 200 to 400 percent increased risk of heart disease and markedly increased risk of death. Blockages can build up in the most critical part of a coronary artery in an incredibly short period of time. In fact, if you're young and healthy, you may have completely clean, smooth, open coronary arteries except for one juncture. In a very close friend of mine, that's exactly what happened. That blockage of a branch of his left coronary artery killed him within hours. He had no warning, no symptoms, no reason to be concerned. In fact, he had only the most modest elevations of blood sugar and cholesterol.

For diabetics, the lower the cholesterol the better is the watchword. Your bad (LDL) cholesterol should be below 100. Top academic experts believe that even lower is better and advise their patients to bring their LDL down to 60: Diabetics have the additional complication of having high levels of triglycerides and lower levels of good (HDL) cholesterol. Diabetics may need to be on combination therapy: statins for their LDL and fibrates for their triglycerides.

Women. Although the most common cause of death in women is heart disease, women have been underrepresented in drug trials and so less information is known about the proper treatment. Women are also less likely to be diagnosed or treated for their heart disease. As you've seen, symptoms tend to be atypical. In my mother's case, even though she had already had a heart attack documented on an EKG, doctors didn't prescribe even the most routine preventive medications. It was not until she was eighty-nine that I convinced her to take statins. For husbands, sons, and daughters, the undertreatment of women with heart disease is a national tragedy. The National Institutes of Health has addressed the problem and there are trials underway to benefit future generations. Meanwhile, the treatment of women by balloon therapy or surgery has vastly improved.

Older patients. Older people often get far less aggressive treatment than younger patients for everything from chest pain to heart attacks. Ironically, it turns out that older patients actually benefit more than younger patients because they're at higher risk. Here's the math. Proper treatment can save the lives of five older patients with heart disease out of every one hundred, but only 1.5 out of every one hundred younger patients. Doctors are just now beginning to learn to treat older patients more aggressively because they benefit so much more from these interventions. "It used to be said they're too old, don't do it, but it should be just the opposite, they're old, be aggressive," says Dr. Jeffrey Moses of New York's Lenox Hill Hospital.

If your doctor ignores you because you are old or ignores your parents because they're old, remember that at any age, all life is infinitely precious. Remember too that 80 percent of deaths in older people are from cardiovascular disease. Research reported in *The Lancet* in 2002 showed that cholesterol lowering with statins was just as effective for people over seventy as for those in middle age. This flies in the face of what many cardiologists have preached and what the guidelines set forth.

One big reason older patients haven't benefited is that compliance is often poor. "We found that sustained, long-term use of statins in elderly patients is low, with the most rapid decline in use occurring in the first year of treatment," concluded Dr. Jerry Avorn, chief of the division of pharmacoepidemiology and pharmacoeconomics at Brigham and Women's Hospital in *JAMA*.

Who is least likely to continue taking statins? Those who are older, have depression or dementia, and/or are taking many prescription drugs. Several major clinical trials are now underway to further clarify the role of cholesterol lowering in older adults.

Aortic stenosis. The narrowing of the main valve controlling the flow of blood out of the heart's main pumping chamber is a serious and, if left untreated, fatal condition. Studies have given some hope that the use of statins can decrease the inflammation of the valve and slow the narrowing. A new trial, underway in Norway, combines simvastatin with ezetimibe (Zetia) in patients with aortic stenosis.

Dr. James Atkins adds, "Statins have also been shown to improve bone density in animals and in subgroups of humans." Statins may also help stave off stroke and Alzheimer's.

CURRENT GUIDELINES

How low should your cholesterol be? The real question is how much can you lower your LDL cholesterol? These are the recommended goals for LDL cholesterol levels.

- Low Risk: less than 160mg/dL
- Moderate Risk, two-plus risk factors: LDL below 130 mg/dL
- High Risk, known heart disease or a major risk factor, such as diabetes: LDL below 100 mg/dL. Optional goal: 70mg/dL.

These are the most recently updated goals. If you attain these goals, you will lower your risk of disease. The question remains, however, how far below these benchmarks you should aim for.

THE COMING REVOLUTION

The goal with any medication should be to prescribe the lowest dosage that achieves optimal results. Yet many people think that less is always better, as if they are cutting back on desserts or alcohol. This is a mistake: Less medicine equals less benefit—especially with statins, which have such a low incidence of side effects.

Dr. Richard Stein says, "Most of us now believe that the 100 mark ought to be a little lower. And how low is the question. The studies that have shown the best clinical outcomes, the AVERT trial and others, have gotten LDLs down to the 70s by using high doses of atorvastatin or simvastatin."

When you're born, your LDL cholesterol is around 60. Some doctors feel that any value greater than 70 may allow the growth of cholesterol blockages in your coronary arteries. As you've seen, half of all heart attacks occur in people who have cholesterol levels that are considered average or even normal. The cutting edge of medicine would have you get your bad cholesterol as low as possible. "We need about 20 to 60 mg/dL to meet our body's needs; all the rest above these levels may be surplus, and it is this surplus that is causing the epidemic of heart disease in our country," says Dr. James McKenney.

Dr. Steven Nissen suggests that "the lining of the heart's arteries actually begins to deteriorate whenever the LDL gets above about 60 or 65. Young children are growing and making new brain cells, doing everything they need to do with LDL cholesterol at 50 and 60, so we don't think that's necessarily an unhealthy level." What Dr. Nissen is referring to with young children is that you do actually need cholesterol, which is why your body makes it in the first place. However, even at a low level of 50, the body appears to have enough.

Bolstering the less LDL the better argument is an English study of 20,000 high-risk patients that concluded that no matter what level your cholesterol, even if it is below 100, lowering it farther provides additional benefit. Currently the best hint that this strategy may be successful is a study by Dr. Allen Taylor, director of cardiovascular research at the Walter Reed Army Medical Center in Washington, DC. Ultrasound measurements showed that high-dose atorvastatin was more effective than a standard dose of pravastatin in slowing or preventing thickening of the arteries. The differences were in fractions of millimeters, but the data did suggest regression, which would mean reversal of disease. The thickness of the carotid artery actually decreased, from an average of 0.625 mm to an average of 0.591 mm. (Keep in mind that it's very hard to measure accurately.)

Dr. Steven Nissen cautions, "The study is useful and important, but was not blinded, it was an open label study." Dr. Nissen has a new study looking at the coronary arteries themselves, which he hopes to release soon and which shows reversal (lower LDL is better). "If I were a betting man," he says, "I'd bet almost anything and even give you odds that reversal will be strongly positive." Dr. Michael Clearfield, associate dean for clinical research at the University of North Texas Health Science Center, concludes, "It's my guess that if we could magically have everyone in this country keep LDL at 100 or less for his or her life span, within a generation heart disease would no longer be the number one killer."

Three major trials are looking at average levels and very low levels to see if LDL of 70 is better in terms of actually reducing heart disease and death compared to just bringing LDL down to 100. These trials are going to change the way we treat patients, predicts Dr. James McKenney.

Consult your doctor to decide whether it makes sense to preempt these studies and begin a much more aggressive statin treatment now. If on the list on page 145 you have a large risk of side effects and your risk of heart disease is low, you may want to wait.

Tragically, many of those at the very highest risk are not

getting treated at all, according to Dr. Luther Clark. Those include patients who have already had a heart attack and even have type 2 diabetes. As you've seen, diabetics have a marked increase risk of heart attack and need to be treated aggressively. They're not on treatment either because it hasn't been recognized that they are at high risk, or drugs have been recommended but they are not taking them. These are the patients most likely to benefit. Others missed time and again are those with a strong family history of heart disease. Many of these people can be fatalistic. But the fact is that a family history is not an automatic death sentence.

THE RIGHT DOSE FOR YOU

Despite the promise of ever better results, most patients taking statins don't achieve their goals. They begin taking too low a dose and that dose is never raised. Let's take an example. Say your LDL cholesterol is 200 mg/dL and your goal is 100 mg/dL. Large starting doses would be required: 40 mg of atorvastatin or 80 mg of simvastatin. Many doctors, fearful of side effects, start low and stay low. What should you do?

Results have their maximum effect after four to six weeks. Between six and eight weeks, your doctor should order a cholesterol panel to determine your LDL cholesterol, HDL cholesterol, and triglycerides while on statins. Later, another measure of your LDL should be taken and both results averaged. This last step is the most important. At this point, your doctor can decide whether you are reaching your goal. Most patients never do. This follow-up visit is critical to your long-term success. Many of us wait for long-term results, rather than monitoring progress (or lack of progress) along the way. One remarkable facet of statins is just how quickly they can work to lower LDL, stabilize blockages, and cut your risk.

EQUIVALENT DOSES

You'll find a bewildering number of cholesterol-lowering agents. Ten mg of one is not equivalent to 10 mg of another. Here is a basic comparison of doses of the leading medications, which will give you the equivalent effect:

10 mg atorvastatin (Lipitor)
20 mg simvastatin (Zocor)
40 mg pravastatin (Pravachol)
40 mg lovastatin (Mevacor, Altocor; Altocor contains nicotinic acid also)
80 mg fluvastatin (Lescol)

STARTING DAILY DOSE

atorvastatin: 10 mg
fluvastatin: 20 mg
lovastatin: 20 mg
pravastatin: 20 mg
rosuvastatin: 5 mg
simvastatin: 20 mg

MAXIMUM DAILY DOSE
APPROVED BY THE FDA

atorvastatin: 80 mg
fluvastatin: 80 mg
lovastatin: 80 mg
pravastatin: 80 mg
rosuvastatin: 40 mg
simvastatin: 80 mg

PREPARATIONS

atorvastatin: 10, 20, 40, 80 mg tablets
fluvastatin: 10, 20, 40, 80 (extended release) mg tablets
lovastatin: 10, 20, 40 mg tablets
pravastatin: 10, 20, 40, 80 mg tablets
rosuvastatin: 5, 10, 20, 40 mg tablets (rosuvastatin was
    approved in August 2003 and has been shown to cut
    LDL by as much as 62 percent in six weeks)
simvastatin: 5, 10, 20, 40, 80 mg tablets

The recent massive ALLHAT study found no difference between statins studied in terms of death rates or heart attacks. However, if you want to go to the most effective doses, at the present time only simvastatin (Zocor) and atorvastatin (Lipitor) get you there. Pravastatin, although less effective at lowering cholesterol to very low levels, proved very effective at reducing heart attack in a variety of studies. In addition, it has fewer side effects because it doesn't require the liver to metabolize it, making it a very safe drug for long-term use and in older and frail patients.

Statins are usually taken in a single dose either with dinner or before bed. This takes advantage of the fact that the body makes more cholesterol at night than during the day. (With longer-acting statins like Atorva, there is no advantage to evening dosing.)

Which drug your doctor chooses may depend on cost. Some insurance plans work out deals with one manufacturer and not with another. If within three months your LDL is not low enough, your doctor may consider switching to a more powerful statin or adding another drug. For instance, he or she might suggest combining a statin with a cholesterol-lowering agent that acts on uptake rather than production (e.g., the bile acid sequestrate Welchol), or with cholestyramine or Zetia.

Statins are seen by many as a single-shot, magic bullet for heart disease. Don't get me wrong, they are amazing. Lowering your risk by 30 percent with just one pill a day is a good start.

Add a healthy lifestyle, aspirin, blood pressure control, or other medications such as beta-blockers, and you've dropped your risk by up to 60 percent. When the new HDL-raising drugs become available (in three to five years), expect even larger decreases in risk. Dr. Steven Nissen would like to see a 50 percent increase in HDL and at least a 50 percent decrease in LDL.

STATIN BOOSTERS

ACE INHIBITORS

In the last five years, ACE inhibitors have come to the fore. They've been used for high blood pressure and heart failure, but now it also looks as if they have a profound effect on people who are at high risk for coronary disease or already have coronary disease. And their effects are additive to that of statins. ACE inhibitors may help slow the progression of heart disease. The bottom line: ACE inhibitors enhance your survival.

Here is a list of ACE inhibitors:

benzapril (Lotensin)
captopril (Capoten)
enalapril (Vasotec)
fosinopril (Monopril)
lisinopril (Zestril, Prinivil)
moexipril (Univasc)
perindopril (Aceon)
quinapril (Accupril)
ramipril (Altace)
trandolapril (Mavik)

How they work. ACE inhibitors stop the production of a chemical that makes blood vessels narrow. By dilating the blood vessels, ACE inhibitors lower blood pressure and reduce the load on the heart for patients with heart failure and may cause beneficial remodeling of the extracellular matrix, the scaffold on which heart muscle cells are arranged for optimal function. They are prescribed after a heart attack to help the heart pump blood better. ACE inhibitors may also help prevent the plaque from fracturing, which is why their lifesaving effect occurs so quickly.

Who should take them. The American Heart Association and American College of Cardiology recommend ACE inhibitors for these conditions:

- A history of heart attack with associated congestive heart failure
- A heart attack damaging the front wall of the heart (an anterior myocardial infarction)
- Dysfunction of the left ventricle, the main pumping chamber of your heart

Recent evidence now suggests that ACE inhibitors should be used in patients who are at high risk for cardiovascular disease even without documented heart failure or high blood pressure. If you are at high risk and looking for an extra edge in your treatment, be sure to discuss ACE inhibitors with your doctor.

Despite the recommendations of the AHA and the ACC, the number of patients receiving ACE inhibitors for these conditions is very small.

Dr. Jeffrey Borer points out that not all ACE inhibitors are created equal. Only ramipril and perindopril have been shown effective in reducing the coronary event—heart attack, angioplasty, bypass surgery, death—rate.

Like statins, ACE inhibitors are emerging as a medication that every patient with heart disease should consider. A recent analysis considered more than thirty studies, including the landmark SOLVD and V-HeFT studies. The authors concluded that ACE inhibitors decreased the risk of death by 23 percent, largely due to fewer deaths from progressive heart failure. "I would put patients on an ACE inhibitor if they have established coronary disease," says Dr. Gary Francis. "That's from the HOPE study. There's less onset of diabetes, there's less stroke, there're fewer coronary events—everything is improved. These drugs are fantastic."

The more recently reported EUROPA study using the drug perindopril in a patient population less sick than in the HOPE study showed similar benefits. Not every physician is impressed with the potential benefits of ACE inhibitors in heart failure. Dr. Steven Nissen is waiting for more persuasive evidence.

The most common side effect is a cough. If it's just a slight cough that's a little bit annoying but you can live with it, continue on the medication. About 5–7 percent of patients on ACE inhibitors find that the cough actually interferes with the quality of their life. In that case, consider an angiotensin reception blocker (ARB).

ANGIOTENSIN RECEPTOR BLOCKERS (ARBS)

If you can't tolerate an ACE inhibitor, consider taking an ARB. (Angiotensin receptor blockers inhibit the effects of angiotensin II at the receptor level and can be used in patients who are intolerant of ACE inhibitors.) ARBs may be considered first-line therapy if you are diabetic and have kidney disease. Researchers are trying to determine if ARBs and ACE inhibitors may be taken together for an even more potent disease preventive effect. While the VALHEFT and CHARM studies have shown effectiveness for improving congestive heart failure, presumptions about the effect on coronary artery disease make sense but are still speculative.

OTHER CHOLESTEROL-LOWERING DRUGS

The vast majority of patients believe that lowering their LDL cholesterol is all that is necessary to prevent a heart attack. In fact, there are other very important blood fats that can increase your risk. For instance, even if your LDL cholesterol is reduced to its goal, your triglyceride level could be high enough to kill you. High triglycerides are associated with coagulation abnormalities, which make it easier for your blood to clot. Low levels of good HDL cholesterol also pose a substantial risk.

Consider niacin, resins, fibrates, and fish oil to lower triglycerides, boost HDL, or further lower LDL if statins are not effective enough.

NIACIN

Nicotinic acid (niacin) is a quadruple hitter. It raises your HDL cholesterol by 15 to 30 percent, lowers your LDL cholesterol by 10 to 20 percent, lowers your triglycerides by 20 to 50 percent, and lowers your CRP. This effect on HDL is its most dramatic capability. Your doctor may add niacin to your statin prescription just to raise your good cholesterol. The two are a very potent combination.

In a recent study using simvastatin with niacin, bad cholesterol dropped 42 percent and good cholesterol rose 26 percent. Impressively, the progress of coronary artery disease was slowed, halted, and even reversed. Bad events were decreased by a whopping 60 percent. The niacin-statin combination is the biggest winner in cardiology. Unfortunately, as Dr. Steven Nissen says, lipid-lowering drugs besides statins are very underutilized. "Niacin should probably be used more often. Since it's not profitable for the pharmaceutical industry, it tends not to be heavily marketed. One reason it's not so popular is that you have to use a lot of it. The effective doses start at about 1000 mg and go up from there. Second, both immediate release and slow release tend to cause a certain number of side effects. Flushing is the biggest problem. Men can get to feel like menopausal women—hot flashes. The hot flashes tend to be less of a problem if you're willing to start with a low dose of the drug and slowly and gradually work your way up to higher doses."

The best candidates for niacin fall into two categories:

- Patients who have low HDL even after taking a statin. The newest guidelines call for using combination therapy— statins and niacin, or statins and fibric acid derivatives and niacin—in patients who have high LDLs and low HDLs, says Dr. Richard Stein.
- Patients who can't tolerate statins.

There are three types of nicotinic acid: immediate release, timed release, and extended release. Many experts prefer the immediate-release form. Be sure to have your doctor monitor you for side effects at the higher dose.

Note that the niacin you can buy over the counter may not lower cholesterol. Nicotinamide, another form of the vitamin niacin, does not lower cholesterol levels.

The usual starting dose is 500 mg, increasing to 3000 mg as necessary. Your doctor will want to start with a low daily dose and then gradually increase the dosage level to between 1500 and 3000 mg per day for the immediate-release form and 1500 and 2000 mg per day for the other forms. Dr. Steven

Nissen says, "I usually start patients at 500 mg taken at bedtime. I strongly prefer the slow-release form because it's less likely to produce flushing. And if you get up to 1500 to 2000 mg a day, you can raise HDL by 25 to 35 percent and lower LDL.

Side Effects. Flushing and hot flashes are the most common side effects, although both usually recede within six to eight weeks. This results from blood vessels opening. If you're still having problems after taking the drug for a while, try taking niacin during or after meals. Try the extended-release form to reduce these side effects as well.

Niacin also may boost the potency of your blood pressure medications, so it's important that your doctor carefully monitors your blood pressure.

The most important side effects are all in the gastrointestinal system: nausea, indigestion, gas, vomiting, diarrhea, the activation of peptic ulcers, liver problems, gout, and high blood sugar. Niacin's effect on blood sugar is potent enough that some doctors avoid using it in diabetics.

Seem like a lot of trouble? It's one big reason that neither doctors nor patients were very keen about taking cholesterol-lowering drugs until the nearly side-effect-free statins came along. However, using the right formulations and beginning at low doses can make them very tolerable.

RESINS

Before the high-tech statins came along and cut cholesterol levels at the site of production, the best idea was to trap the cholesterol in the intestinal tract and prevent it from being reabsorbed into the bloodstream with materials called resins. They work like this: The bile acids, which enter the intestine from the gallbladder, have a high cholesterol content. The intestine uses these acids to help with digestion. Then the intestine actively re-absorbs them into the bloodstream after their job with digestion is completed. Resins (also called bile acid sequestrants) trap the bile acids in the intestine and force them to exit the body in the stool. This lowers cholesterol by as much as 20 percent.

These older drugs are not used much when compared to statins, since they don't share the same cholesterol-lowering power and have more side effects, especially involving the gastrointestinal system. Their major use today is in patients who cannot tolerate statins, or to further lower cholesterol levels when statins aren't enough. Working together, resins and statins can lower LDL cholesterol by more than 40 percent.

Since the absorption of fat-soluble vitamins A, D, E, and K occurs with resin use, be sure to check with your physician about ways to replace those vitamins.

The bile acid sequestrants cholestyramine (Questran), colestipol (Colestid, Lestid), and colesevelam (Welchol) are available as powders or tablets. Thirty years of experience demonstrate that they are safe for long-term use. Welchol is relatively new. Experts say it's the best tolerated of all the resins and so it's beginning to be the one most prescribed. It's effective at lower doses and appears less likely to cause side effects. These are not the drug of choice if you have a high triglyceride level or suffer severe constipation.

How to take resins. Mix powders with water or fruit juice and take with meals. They are usually taken twice a day. To avoid stomach problems (constipation, bloating, nausea, gas), take the tablets with a large glass of water. Since resins can interfere with other medications, don't take them at the same time as other drugs. The best advice is to take your other medications one hour before or six hours after these.

EZETIMIBE (ZETIA)

Zetia is a new drug approved by the FDA in late 2002. Like resins, zetia blocks cholesterol absorption, but it does so by a completely different mechanism and is much better tolerated. Dr. Steven Nissen says that it tends to boost the efficacy of statins to lower your cholesterol: "Given with a little bit of Zocor makes it act like a lot of Zocor." Dr. Nissen is in the process of designing a clinical trial to test the efficacy of this drug. To summarize, both niacin and resin drugs can boost the effect of statins.

FIBRATES

If you're already taking a statin and have either high triglycerides or low HDL, fibrates may be added.

Fenofibrate (Tricor) and gemfibrozil (Lopid) don't lower LDL cholesterol very much, but they do a great job at lowering triglycerides and raising HDL, something that statins don't do very well. "The idea is, suppose you get put on statins and your LDL comes down but your triglycerides are still high. What are you going to do?" asks Dr. Steven Nissen. Most doctors, he says, don't do anything. "Because the LDL was reduced, they think they've done their job." However, Dr. Nissen says, "The doctors who really get it are the ones who say, 'Gee, your triglycerides are still 250 or 300, I'm going to add fenofibrate and get them down by 30 to 40 percent.' So if statins alone don't do the job, there's an important role for these drugs. Gemfibrozil in the Health Safety study showed a near equal reduction in heart risk as the statins."

Dr. Gary Francis prefers fenofibrate. "I think it's safer than gemfibrozil. The consumer needs to know that gemfibrozil will interact with statins. And there's far more muscle destruction with that combination than there is with, say, a statin alone. There's less interaction, we think, with fenofibrate and a statin."

Since fenofibrate tends to lower triglycerides and raise HDL, it's very good for people with metabolic syndrome or who have a middle-aged spread.

What is remarkable about gemfibrozil is that it reduces the risk of heart attack at a rate nearly equal to that of statins. It drops triglycerides from 20 to 50 percent while HDL cholesterol typically increases 10 to 15 percent. That potent combination decreases heart attack by 22 percent. But since gemfibrozil is not very effective at lowering your LDL cholesterol, you'll still require other medications if your LDL needs to be significantly lowered.

Fibrates are taken two times a day thirty minutes before breakfast and dinner.

Side Effects. You may experience trouble in your gastrointestinal tract and are at a higher risk of developing cholesterol gallstones. Since fibrates may increase the potency of blood thinners, your doctor needs to monitor your blood more carefully if you are taking Coumadin or other blood thinners.

FISH OIL

Fish oil is very important and getting more important all the time, says Dr. Steven Nissen. High-dose fish oil (three capsules three times a day) can lower triglycerides by up to 40–50 percent and it's a natural product. I take a supplement called Eskimo-3, which dissolves in the small intestine, not the stomach, to prevent the bad breath that can result from taking fish oil.

Note: Fish oil is sold over the counter and is safe. Still, tell your doctor if you decide to take it. I can't stress enough the importance of sharing *all* information with *all* of your doctors.

RAISING HDL

HDL cholesterol is notoriously hard to raise, yet a high level is very protective. HDL clears cholesterol out of the artery walls and carries it back to the liver. Statins typically raise HDL as much as 8 percent; niacin might get you up 15 percent. The fibrates gemfibrozil and fenofibrate can raise HDL especially if your triglycerides are high, says Dr. Roger Blumenthal. Weight loss and increased exercise can also raise HDL, though relatively modestly. "HDL isn't talked about a lot because we don't have as many good ways to raise it," continues Dr. Blumenthal. For people with peripheral arterial disease and calf pain with walking (intermittent claudication), cilostazol (Pletal) may provide additional benefits: The drug increases HDL by at least 15 percent.

SUPER HDL

Raising HDL has become the new big idea behind many current drug trials. The hottest new up-and-coming drug is almost like liquid Drano in its ability to clean out coronary arteries. It is a synthetic form of HDL based on a protein called ApoA-I Milano mentioned at the beginning of this book. According to the American Heart Association, "Italian researchers found that 40 residents there [Limone Sul Gardia, Italy] had very low HDL levels, yet paradoxically had low rates of coronary artery disease. Lab tests revealed a likely explanation: All had a gene variation in a key protein component of HDL. The variation contributed to larger-than-normal HDL particles, which is believed to make HDL cholesterol especially efficient at removing plaque." The mutant gene produces particularly efficient HDL. In mice and rats, this mutant HDL removed most of the plaque from their coronary arteries. "At six weeks, imaging tests showed the patients receiving the synthetic protein had a visible 4 percent reduction in plaque buildup in their coronary arteries." This was first used on very sick patients with unstable angina.

Says Dr. Steven Nissen, an author of the study, "The study was positive and the stock on Wall Street went nuts. So we gave this mutant HDL to patients and we actually reversed their disease. I almost fell off my seat. I really didn't think the study was going to be positive—it was just too small and too quick." Time will tell if these results translate directly to clinical benefits.

In another study, an HDL-raising drug was delivered as a vaccine to stimulate the immune system to block a protein involved in cholesterol transfer.

Just how important is HDL? Dr. James Atkins says that patients who have very high HDL cholesterol, above 75, live five to seven years longer than others and rarely have coronary artery disease despite their diet, and even smoking. At the opposite end of the scale, people with very low HDL cholesterol (20) are almost sure to develop heart disease even with the best prevention.

DRUGS THAT LOWER HIGH BLOOD PRESSURE

Fatal Flaw

A friend of mine called me in a panic last year. Her father had suffered a massive stroke. I spoke with her father's doctor, who wanted to suspend all but supportive treatment; the man appeared doomed to die. What happened? His physician had diagnosed his hypertension and had prescribed the right medications. But like too many patients, my friend's father rarely took the right amount of the correct medication at the right time. He paid a terrible price.

If you're taking medication, make certain you take the right amount at the right time. Too many patients think that just as long as they take some medication some of the time, they'll be fine. Many turn out dead wrong. Dr. Paul Whelton of the Tulane University Health Sciences Center says that "those who are aware of their high blood pressure either aren't treated or are inadequately treated." In fact, in the United States, only about one-third of hypertensives are being controlled to the recommended blood pressure levels, says Dr. Claude Lenfant. Since hypertension is so common, people don't take it seriously enough.

HIGH BLOOD PRESSURE

High blood pressure is a separate disease from coronary artery disease. It's included here because a high blood pressure combined with high cholesterol increases your risk of a heart attack. Inversely, adding a blood-pressure-lowering drug to a cholesterol-lowering drug can decrease the likelihood you'll have a heart attack.

High blood pressure is a stand-alone major risk factor for heart disease even if you have a normal or even low cholesterol. The best drug for lowering blood pressure in patients with heart disease isn't clearly defined. While low-dose thiazide diuretics and beta-blockers remain first-line agents, ACE inhibitors and ARBs might be considered first line in patients with known heart disease or with particularly high levels of the hormone renin, which causes the body to produce chemicals that narrow the arterioles and raise blood pressure. Additional blood pressure medications should be added as needed to reach the target blood pressure.

There are 50 million Americans with hypertension, but only about 70 percent are aware they have the condition, just 59 percent get treated, and only 34 percent are able to lower their blood pressure to 140/90.

Blood pressure control has fallen into the dullest backwater of preventive medicine. Statins are the biggest, brightest star because the side effects are so few and the results so brilliant. Blood pressure medications can have side effects, and many are not dramatic in their effectiveness. For those reasons, patient compliance is deplorable. Unfortunately, that means tens of thousands of Americans pay the ultimate price every year, suffering heart attacks, debilitating strokes, and sudden death.

The NHLBI estimates that one of every two adults over the age of sixty has high blood pressure. Blood pressure increases as you age. As you go from middle to old age, there is a 90 percent chance you'll develop high blood pressure, and that increases your chance of a heart attack.

As your blood pressure slowly sneaks up, there is a tendency to ignore it, figuring that it's always been normal so it will be okay now. High normal is a systolic of 130–139 mmHg and a diastolic of 85–89 mmHg. If you are in the high normal range, your risk of a bad event or death within ten years is up to two and half times higher than those with optimal blood pressure, which is considered less than 120 systolic and less than 80 diastolic. Just to drive the point home, at age fifty-five, even with normal blood pressure, your lifetime risk of developing hypertension is 90 percent.

DETERMINING YOUR BLOOD PRESSURE

When your doctor listens to the sounds in your arteries through a stethoscope while the blood pressure cuff is released, he or she hears two sounds. The first is called the systolic blood pressure, the higher number. A systolic blood pressure at or above 140 mmHg is high. When the sound of your beating heart heard through the stethoscope placed on an artery in your arm fades, your doctor records a second number, the diastolic blood pressure. If your diastolic blood pressure is at or above 90 mmHg, you have high blood pressure. It's also important to have two measures taken and then averaged after you've been sitting quietly for five minutes to get a better reading. Home monitors are becoming increasingly popular.

People always ask me what their blood pressure should be. The Joint National Committee on Detection, Evaluation, and Diagnosis of High Blood Pressure recommends that if you already have heart disease, your blood pressure should be lowered to below 130/85 mmHg. Just as diabetics need to have lower cholesterol, they also need to have lower blood pressure than the general public, below 130/80. If diabetics have protein in their urine (> 1 g/dL of proteinuria), their blood pressure should be less than 125/75 mmHg.

WHEN SHOULD YOU START ON MEDICATION?

Even if you don't have heart disease or diabetes, consider improving your diet and getting more exercise if your systolic blood pressure is greater than 160 mmHg or your diastolic is greater than 100 mmHg. If, after six months, diet and exercise don't bring you down to the established target of less than 140/90 mmHg, consider taking medications.

What's the right diet? While there are many, Dr. Paul Whelton recommends an Asian diet. "We know very well that certain dietary approaches, particularly care with weight, moderation of sodium intake, higher potassium, and moderation of alcohol intake, can lower blood pressure. The DASH (Dietary Approaches to Stop Hypertension) diet is basically an Eastern-type diet high in fruits, vegetables, and low-fat dairy products. It's a very effective diet in preventing and lowering high blood pressure." The DASH diet is particularly high in foods that contain potassium, calcium, and magnesium; together with minimizing (not eliminating) sodium (an essential element for life), enhancement of these elements is thought to be the basis of the diet's effectiveness.

Dr. Whelton emphasizes that "the other thing we know with great certainty is that aerobic exercise will prevent and lower blood pressure." It doesn't have to be high intensity, but it does need to be fairly consistent. You can learn more about the DASH diet at the NHLBI's Web site (www.nhlbi.nih.gov).

What are the rewards of lowering blood pressure? A 27 percent decreased risk of heart attack, a 37 percent decreased risk of stroke, and a stunning 55 percent decreased risk of heart failure.

Systolic blood pressure is becoming the principal clinical indicator for the detection, evaluation, and treatment of hypertension, especially in middle-aged and older Americans. Major epidemiologic research shows that death and disability from heart disease increase in direct proportion to systolic blood pressure across a very wide range of blood pressures. High systolic pressure is also incredibly common. Treating isolated systolic hypertension reduces stroke, heart attack, heart failure, kidney failure, and overall death and disability from heart disease.

Ironically, as important as systolic hypertension is, even with aggressive management systolic blood pressure is less well controlled than diastolic. In the MRFIT and HOT trials, diastolic control exceeded 90 percent, but systolic control was less than 60 percent. From the earliest days of these major blood pressure studies, systolic blood pressure has been a strong cardiovascular disease risk factor.

Just to drive the point home, systolic hypertension is the most prevalent risk factor for heart failure and interacts with both high cholesterol and diabetes. As you age, systolic blood pressure is the one you have to worry about most. While diastolic declines over age fifty-five, systolic steadily increases.

A final reason for focusing on systolic blood pressure: The diagnosis is far more accurate than diastolic. In the famous Framingham study, 91 percent of systolic high blood pressure was correctly classified and only 22 percent of diastolic.

OLDER PATIENTS

Just because blood pressure rises as we age doesn't mean it's okay. Older patients are already especially prone to undertreatment. For instance, over the age of seventy, only 25 percent of African Americans and 18 percent of white Americans achieve the blood pressure goals recommended to them. And when African Americans do take certain drugs, such as ACE inhibitors, they do not work as well, says Dr. Steven Nissen.

You may want to consider ACE inhibitors, which carry a lower complication and death rate for older patients. Be cautious, however, if you have long-standing severe systolic hypertension; rapid lowering of your blood pressure could prove harmful. If you fit into this category or if your blood pressure is brittle (subject to sharp rises and drops) or resistant to treatment, you need to lower your blood pressure more slowly. Ultimately, however, your goal is to get as close to your target blood pressure as possible. In fact, gradual control of blood pressure not only is a good idea but also is what happens when any antihypertensive drug is given: It takes at least two weeks of treatment with a single-dose regimen to achieve 90 percent of the blood pressure lowering you will eventually achieve with that dose. Most hypertension specialists believe that it takes at least six weeks, and often longer, to see the complete effect of a single drug at a single dose. Therefore, frequent upward titration of dose, and addition of new drugs, probably is not a good idea unless your blood pressure is in the severe range or is malignant, that is, associated with evidence of acute organ damage.

BLOOD PRESSURE MEDICATIONS

DIURETICS

Also called water pills because they flush excess water and sodium from the body, these are dirt-cheap, simple medications. Their sales have been steadily declining from 56 percent of blood pressure prescriptions in 1982 to 27 percent in 1992, as manufacturers promote newer, more expensive drugs. However, the major new ALLHAT study demonstrated that, predominantly in relatively older patients with systolic hypertension, a common diuretic called chlorthalidone was superior at preventing major events from cardiovascular disease compared to each of the major treatment drugs studied: a calcium channel blocker, an ACE inhibitor, and an alpha-adrenergic blocker. Most recent research compared new medications to a placebo. ALLHAT provided a head-to-head competition, which had been long awaited by physicians. A diuretic could cost as little as $25 a year, compared to $250 for an ACE inhibitor or $500 for a calcium channel blocker. The study's author, Dr. Paul Whelton, points out that there is a "lot less" heart failure found in patients taking diuretics than in the other drug treatment groups. Dr. Steven Nissen is not as enthusiastic; he says there is slightly less heart failure.

The diuretic group also achieved slightly better blood pressure control. The superiority of diuretics in preventing major forms of heart disease, and their lower cost, makes them drugs of first choice in beginning the treatment of hypertension for many.

If you can't tolerate a diuretic or, for other reasons, your doctor believes a different type of drug is appropriate for your particular situation, he or she may consider ACE inhibitors, calcium channel blockers, or beta-blockers (alpha-blockers aren't usually considered for initial therapy). Remember, you're looking for a twofer: great control of your blood pressure and protection from heart disease. You may well end up on one of these other medications in addition to your diuretic since most patients with high blood pressure require more than one medication plus solid lifestyle changes. What if you're already taking another medication? The authors of ALLHAT suggest considering a change to a thiazide, even if you are well controlled. As always, consider this change carefully with your physician.

ACE INHIBITORS

You've seen how effective these drugs are for preventing heart disease in people without hypertension. Now the HOPE and EUROPA studies support the use of ACE inhibitors as first-line drugs for hypertensive patients with heart disease or diabetes. There was a 27 percent lower incidence of heart attack and death in those treated with an ACE inhibitor in the HOPE trial, and a similar reduction in EUROPA.

Angiotensin converting enzyme (ACE) inhibitors prevent the formation of a hormone called angiotensin II, which normally causes blood vessels to narrow. The ACE inhibitors cause the vessels to relax, and blood pressure goes down.

BETA-BLOCKERS

Beta-blockers are another starter medication if you've never been treated for hypertension before. Beta-blockers can be added to other medications such as diuretics for more effective control, especially if you're younger than age sixty. Since beta-blockers can block the effect of insulin and can restrict blood flow, you may want to avoid them if you have diabetes or peripheral artery disease. Beta-blockers also have other powerful life-extending benefits if you have already had a heart attack or have heart failure. Receiving a beta-blocker during a heart attack can reduce both acute and long-term risk of death up to 35 percent. Dr. Paul Whelton advises, "Beta-blockers are the best proven drug to reduce risk after a heart attack."

The downside is that beta-blockers are associated with sexual dysfunction and depression in some individuals. They may also cause airway narrowing in asthmatics. "The key is to start with a very low dose and gradually titrate up. Because if you start with a big dose, invariably patients don't seem to like them. They're tired, men get erectile dysfunction, everyone just complains. So start with a low dose and then gradually (by gradually I mean like every two weeks or so) increase the dose, and then the tolerability goes way up," advises Dr. Gary Francis.

CALCIUM CHANNEL BLOCKERS (CCBS)

Both the SHEP and Syst-EUR studies recommend long-acting calcium channel blockers for isolated systolic high blood pressure; doctors often use CCBs along with a diuretic. It is important to know that there are three different types of drugs called calcium channel blockers, and their optimal applications are different. In their long-acting forms, all can lower blood pressure and prevent angina; only some are useful in acute coronary events like unstable angina (acute coronary syndrome) or heart attack.

Calcium channel blockers prevent calcium from entering the muscle cells of the heart and blood vessels, causing blood vessels to relax and blood pressure to go down.

If you have chest pain from heart disease, your doctor may give you a calcium channel blocker. Some are also used after an acute heart attack. "In all other circumstances I would say a diuretic should be the starting drug because it's very well proven and very inexpensive, and it's sort of the base upon which everything else would be used," says Dr. Paul Whelton. Dr. Gary

Francis says that calcium channel blockers have the best record of preventing stroke of all antihypertensives. "That's their main virtue. The kind of patients we see almost never could be controlled on one drug. Often diabetics may require five to seven drugs. CCBs are add-on drugs. They do control blood pressure and are effective, but they're expensive."

Not all physicians are big fans of CCBs. Dr. James Atkins discourages their use because "calcium channel blockers do not improve life expectancy and they may actually in a few patients do some harm, whereas beta-blockers have a protective benefit." Bottom line, you want a first-line drug that may improve your longevity. If you take beta-blockers during an acute heart attack, you may reduce both your immediate acute and long-term mortality between 25 and 35 percent. "Calcium channel blockers are either neutral or carry a 4 percent increase in mortality in certain high-risk individuals," says Dr. Atkins. "A calcium channel blocker in someone who has heart failure is not protective at all and tends to cause slight harm." My father was on a calcium channel blocker when he died. He had heart failure, and I had warned his cardiologist.

Asthmatics, who can't use beta-blockers because of their effect on the airways, are candidates for calcium channel blockers. In asthmatics, "you're forced to use a calcium channel blocker and you realize it's nowhere near as effective at preventing a subsequent heart attack or sudden death," says Dr. James Atkins.

Calcium channel blockers can be excellent add-on drugs if your first-line choice, such as diuretics, is not totally effective and you require further medication. Some calcium channel blockers (verapamil and diltiazem) can also be used for controlling heart rate in patients with atrial fibrillation, though other choices exist and may be more appropriate in many settings.

OTHER DRUGS

The following classes of medication are used to treat complex and difficult cases of hypertension. If you have exhausted the benefits of the above drugs and require the addition of these drugs, you should be at a center that specializes in hypertension.

- **Vasodilators:** decrease blood pressure by relaxing the muscle in blood vessel walls and allowing the vessels to dilate.
- **Nervous system inhibitors:** lower blood pressure by inhibiting nerve impulses, which contract blood vessels. This allows blood vessels to dilate, thereby reducing pressure.
- **Alpha-blockers:** According to results from an NHLBI clinical study, an alpha-blocker may not be the best choice for initial treatment of uncomplicated high blood pressure. The ALLHAT study stopped the use of these drugs early on because of the substantially higher rate of problems, including twice the rate of hospitalization for heart failure. And the 25 percent increase in cardiovascular events was precisely what patients were trying to prevent.
- **Alpha-beta blockers:** work the same way as alpha-blockers but also slow the heartbeat, as beta-blockers do. As a result, less blood is pumped through the vessels and the blood pressure goes down.
- **Angiotensin antagonists:** a relatively new type of high blood pressure drug that shields blood vessels from angiotensin II. As a result, the vessels become wider and blood pressure goes down.

How low should your blood pressure be? In theory, the lower the better, just like cholesterol. Two important trials show marked benefit to getting your systolic below 160. Is even lower better?

The perindopril/indapamide study analyzed patients whose blood pressure was within the normal range and found a reduction in strokes when their blood pressure was further lowered. To protect your brain, kidneys, and heart from damage, lifelong maintenance below 140/90 is the goal. "This is the standard, but a lot of us think that the lower the better," says Dr. Steven Nissen. "No one's really ever done the trials, but the data are accumulating. I should say it probably doesn't hurt to be even lower." Epidemiological data indicate an increase in cardiovascular events when blood pressure rises above 115/75, and actuarial data (used by insurance companies to define their rates) suggest an increase in events when blood pressure increases above 100/60.

If you have diabetes, your blood pressure should be below 130/85. If you have kidney or heart failure, you should try to reduce your blood pressure to the lowest level possible since you already have organ damage.

If you are not achieving your goals or have excessive side effects from medication, consider going to a center that specializes in hypertension. These centers have an amazing store of experience with which to handle even the toughest problem patients. Managing hypertension can become very complex, with multiple medications required to achieve satisfactory results.

LIFESTYLE THERAPY

Blood pressure often can be brought back into the normal range with lifestyle changes alone. These are not just side effect–free but also make you feel terrific!

The general guidelines are as follows:

- Consume more than 3500 mg of dietary potassium per day. (Good sources are bananas and apricots).
- Eat five to nine servings of fruits and vegetables daily.

- Choose dairy products with reduced saturated and to-tal fat.
- Limit sodium to fewer than 2400 mg (about 1 teaspoon of salt) a day. The best way to do that is by limiting the salt you add to food. Three-fourths of your total intake of salt comes from sodium added during processing and manu-facturing.
- Limit your consumption of alcohol to no more than 24 ounces of beer, ten ounces of wine, or two ounces of 100-proof whiskey per day in men and half that amount in women.
- Lose weight. Even a loss of eight pounds significantly low-ers systolic blood pressure.
- Exercise more. Regular physical activity lowers systolic blood pressure by more than 4 mmHg.

DRUGS THAT TREAT CORONARY ARTERY DISEASE

Most of this chapter has been devoted to the slowing, preven-tion, or outright reversal of coronary artery disease. If you al-ready have symptomatic coronary artery disease, below are the medications you should review with your cardiologist. In Step 7, "Get the Right Lifesaving Procedure," you'll see that one key criterion for balloon therapy or bypass surgery is failure of med-ical therapy.

Here I describe the medical therapy you should try first. You'll note that the beginning of this list includes exactly the same preventive drugs we just looked at, and for good reason. They are aimed at the underlying disease process. Many also have proven benefits in terms of preventing heart attacks and death. You can think of them as dual-purpose medications.

There is a tremendous allure to having a procedure done because of the quick-fix nature, but proper medical therapy, in the right circumstance, can have a tremendous long-lasting effect.

LIPID-LOWERING DRUGS

These are statins and niacin. Since you have known heart disease, your goals are vastly different from those of patients at lower risk. You should lower your LDL well below 100, even below 60.

Be sure to check your cholesterol two months after a heart attack. Dr. James Atkins counsels that the heart attack itself will lower your LDL cholesterol, as will the diet in the hospital, and your own adrenaline that is pouring out. But this artificial lowering doesn't last. "Here's a very typical example: A patient is discharged on 20 mg of simvastatin, and in a month I bump it to 40, and in two months I bump it to 80, because the LDL continues to climb."

ANTIHYPERTENSIVE DRUGS

These are indicated if you also have high blood pressure.

ANTIPLATELET DRUGS

These are aspirin and clopidogrel. Aspirin is highly recommended for patients who have known heart disease. The addition of clopidogrel may provide an increased antiplatelet effect. This is especially important if you are recovering from a recent acute coronary event (unstable angina, recent heart attack) or have had a stent placed during balloon therapy (described in the next chapter). Whereas the use of aspirin is debatable for those at low risk, it's a must for most patients who have known symptomatic disease.

BETA-BLOCKERS

You've learned how beta-blockers can lower blood pressure. They are also used to prevent chest pain. Here's how. Beta-blockers slow the heart so it does less work, requiring less blood flow in the coronary arteries. Beta-blockers prevent the rise in heart rate with exercise, limiting blood flow requirements. Beta-blockers directly reduce the force of contraction of the heart, lowering oxygen requirement, and may lower blood pressure, also reducing the heart's oxygen demand. If you have chest pain, you're a great candidate for beta-blockers.

Doctors use them routinely after a heart attack because studies have demonstrated that they lower the risk of death. Immediately after a heart attack, beta-blockers can be lifesaving, although they have not been shown to prevent death caused by an irregular heart rhythm (arrhythmia). Dr. James Atkins says, "If you give beta-blockers to an acute MI, you reduce both acute and long-term mortality between 25 and 35 percent."

Beta-blockers have been around forever, yet tragically, the majority of patients who should be taking them are not. I tried for more than a year to have my father put on a beta-blocker. Don't dismiss beta-blockers just because they don't have the dazzle of statins. If you've had a heart attack, you can reduce your risk of another as much with a beta-blocker as you can by lowering your cholesterol.

There are excellent studies showing that beta-blockers are of even greater benefit if your heart is not working up to par, as measured by a lowered ejection fraction. Recently, carvedilol (Coreg), a beta-blocker with additional alpha-blocking activity, has been shown to improve survival after heart attack even in people who also have heart failure or a very low ejection fraction. Such people have a particularly high risk if untreated.

Dr. James Atkins advises, "You should think about beta-blockers in anyone who has atherosclerosis. It is a protective drug. We've proved it post–heart attack; we have very good trials to show that it has a major survival benefit."

The most commonly used beta-blocker after heart attack in patients without heart failure is metoprolol (Lopressor), though several others also have been shown to be effective. This is the best measure of how long these drugs stay in your system:

atenolol: 7–9 hours
metoprolol: 5–6 hours (slow-release Toprol XL lasts up to
   24 hours)
nadolol: 15 hours
propranolol: 3–4 hours

There are newer drugs in the offing that, unlike beta-blockers, have an effect on heart rate only, without the other effects of beta-blockers. Dr. Jeffrey Borer, the author of the published report on the first large trial with such an agent, says it is very impressive for prevention of angina, though effects on subsequent heart attacks or death are not yet known.

LONG-ACTING NITROGLYCERIN FORMULATIONS

The nitroglycerin tablet you put under your tongue lasts for up to two hours when taken to relieve acute chest pain, though maximal effect is somewhat shorter. Long-acting oral preparations prevent chest pain for at least three to five hours, while the transdermal preparations, applied to the skin, act for ten to fourteen hours. The most common longer-duration medication is isosorbide mononitrate (Imdur); an older, and still used, form is isosorbide dinitrate (Isordil).

Note: You want to get ahead of your chest pain by taking nitro before the pain begins, such as before exercise.

CALCIUM CHANNEL BLOCKERS

One key strategy in decreasing chest pain is reducing the work the heart has to do. Calcium channel blockers dilate the arteries and lower the blood pressure, so when the heart pumps it encounters a lower load to pump against. This lessens the need for blood flow through a narrowed coronary artery by reducing the amount of work the heart muscle has to do, thereby decreasing the chest pain.

The three different groups of calcium channel blockers are dihydropyridine, verapamil, and diltiazem. The cleverest part of using CCBs is that you can customize their effect depending on the kind you use. Dr. Jeffrey Borer lays out the strategies:

- The dihydropyridine CCBs are primarily used to dilate blood vessels, which makes them superior for patients with high blood pressure.
     amlodipine (Norvasc) (the most commonly used)
     felodipine (Plendil)
     nicardipine (Cardene, Cardene SR)
     nifedipine (Adalat, Adalat CC, Procardia, Procardia XL)
     nisoldipine (Sular)
- The verapamil group has an important heart-rate-slowing effect as well as some vasodilation action. The heart rate effect lessens the load on the heart to decrease chest pain. It also can be used to decrease the heart rate in conditions

where the rate is dangerously fast, such as for atrial fibrillation.

> Calan, Calan SR, Covera-HS, Isoptin, Isoptin SR, Verelan, Verelan PM

- Diltiazem has features of both vasodilation and rate slowing.

> Cardizem, Cardizem CD, Cardizem SR, Dilacor XR, Diltia XT, Tiazac

As you've seen, after a heart attack, calcium channel blockers are either neutral or carry a 4 percent increase in mortality in certain high-risk individuals, though one study showed a reduction in mortality when verapamil is begun two weeks after a heart attack in patients without heart failure. Be certain to review your risk status before beginning therapy with CCBs.

ACE INHIBITORS

The HOPE trial showed substantial reduction in the risk of heart attack and stroke in patients with known heart disease who are fifty-five or older and who have at least one additional cardiac risk factor, such as high cholesterol, diabetes, or high blood pressure. Only 40 percent of these patients take ACE inhibitors, with tragic consequences. The EUROPA trial recently extended these benefits to patients with known coronary artery disease without risk factors when the ACE inhibitor perindopril is used.

The dose of ACE inhibitors is increased until your goal of therapy is met. ACE inhibitors are not antianginal drugs, but it is possible that, with long-term use, angina frequency might be reduced, though this never has been studied. If you're using ACE inhibitors for high blood pressure, increase the dose until you've adequately treated the high blood pressure without getting unacceptable side effects. If you're using them to prevent bad events after a heart attack, however, the dose isn't really known because clinical trials after heart attacks generally used only one dose, and only two drugs (ramipril and perindopril) have been studied for event reduction irrespective of prior heart attack. Most cardiologists believe that every heart disease patient should consider an ACE inhibitor.

Ramipril (10 mg per day) and perindopril (8 mg per day) have been shown to reduce heart attack plus death risk by more than 20 percent in patients with coronary artery disease. It is possible that other ACE inhibitors have the same benefit, but that isn't known. Dr. Steven Nissen's opinion, however, is that there is "too much hype about HOPE. Ramipiril is *much* more expensive and one of the least effective ACE inhibitors for blood pressure reduction."

DRUGS THAT TREAT CONGESTIVE HEART FAILURE

Patients who have suffered a large heart attack or have had multiple smaller ones or have had failed balloon therapy may end up with so much damaged heart muscle that the heart no longer pumps effectively. To compensate, the heart dilates as pressure backs up, and fluid begins to leak into the lungs.

If you have congestive heart failure, the right drugs make an amazing difference. First, you'll get major symptomatic relief with diuretic drugs like Lasix. Second, you can substantially cut the rather large risk of death (both sudden and pump failure) with drugs like ACE inhibitors, some beta-blockers (carvedilol, metoprolol, and bucindolol), and blockers of aldosterone effect (spironolactone, eplerinone).

Below are the medications you should consider with your doctor. Keep in mind that only these three types of drugs have a real survival benefit. The others, such as digitalis and other diuretics, are for pure symptom relief and do not increase survival.

How do you know if you're headed for congestive heart failure? The easiest way is with an echocardiogram, an essential part of the workup of coronary artery disease. The key measurement you are looking for is ejection fraction. If this has declined substantially, you may benefit from these measures.

BETA-BLOCKERS

It may appear counterintuitive to use beta-blockers with congestive heart failure since they weaken the heart's ability to pump. However, recent studies have shown that judicious amounts, increased very gradually over time, reduce the death rate (both that occurring suddenly and the more gradual death caused by pump dysfunction associated with heart failure). You should ask a specialist in heart failure about beta-blockers' appropriateness in your case.

Only the beta-blocker carvedilol (Coreg) has been studied in the post–heart attack setting in patients with heart failure. That's not to say that the others don't work, but this is the only drug that's been studied in this particular situation. The other trials of post–heart attack patients excluded people with heart failure and were done years ago. Carvedilol was studied recently in the COPERNICUS trial. Carvedilol was shown to reduce additional heart attacks and prolong life in people who'd had a heart attack and who now had low ejection fractions with and without heart failure.

Dr. James Atkins adds metoprolol to carvedilol as a beta-blocker, which has a survival benefit in people with heart failure. Dr. Jeffrey Borer elaborates, "Only metoprolol has been approved for treatment of patients with heart failure and, separately, for patients who have had recent MI without heart failure. Only carvedilol has been studied, and approved, both for patients with heart failure without recent heart attack and for patients with recent MI together with heart failure. The labels of the drugs reflect these differences. It is not advisable to advocate 'off-label' use of metoprolol—for example, for patients with acute MI and heart failure. Moreover, strictly speaking, three beta-blockers, not just two, have been found beneficial for heart failure in the nonacute MI setting: carvedilol, metoprolol, and bucindolol."

ACE INHIBITORS

As you saw above, ACE inhibitors cut the risk of death in people who have had a heart attack and in people with heart failure. If patients can't tolerate ACE inhibitors, doctors use angiotensin receptor blockers for heart failure. Remember, to prevent coronary events, consider the ACE inhibitor ramipril or perindopril.

ACE inhibitors may be one of the most amazing drugs in cardiology because they can affect the shape of the heart. The heart is normally elliptical in shape. After a heart attack, the heart tends to become more rounded. A rounder heart is not nearly as efficient, and a lot more stress is placed on the walls, which leads to more complications and deterioration of function. If very early during an MI you are given an ACE inhibitor, your heart tends to stay elliptical. Could you still change the shape of your heart *after* the damage is done? Yes. After it's become round or globular, ACE inhibitors can remodel it back to being elliptical again, says Dr. James Atkins. Keeping the heart in its normal shape is critical to maintaining excellent function and preventing further deterioration.

DIURETICS

Commonly referred to as water pills, these are used for symptomatic relief of congestive heart failure. Some are more potent (and shorter acting) than the diuretics used for the initial treatment of hypertension, though the diuretics used for hypertension can be used for maintenance treatment of patients with heart failure too.

In heart failure, the body accumulates excess fluid. Diuretics help to remove that fluid and decrease respiratory problems due to water retained in the lungs. Furosemide (Lasix) is the diuretic most frequently used get rid of the excess salt and water. Some people can control their fluids by just cutting down the salt they eat; others need a diuretic.

Spironolactone and eplerinone are the only diuretics that clearly increase survival in patients with heart failure, and they also can be used for hypertension. However, these drugs have the potential disadvantage of retarding potassium excretion by the kidneys. This is an uncommon but potentially serious problem—a very high potassium level in the blood can cause a lethal arrhythmia. Therefore, your potassium level must be carefully monitored if you are taking spironolactone or eplerinone, advises Dr. Jeffrey Borer.

DIGITALIS

Digitalis has been used for seventy years. It helps the heart to beat more forcefully and also acts on the kidneys like a diuretic. Since toxic overdoses may occur, it must be monitored carefully. Digitalis has no survival benefit, but it does reduce symptoms and hospitalizations. Patients have fewer episodes of heart failure and fewer readmissions to the hospital, so it's considered a quality-of-life drug.

ANGIOTENSIN RECEPTOR BLOCKERS

These are an alternative for the 10 to 15 percent of patients who can't tolerate ACE inhibitors because of a chronic cough. ARBs have never been studied specifically for coronary disease, and they are expensive.

SUPPLEMENTS

These are over-the-counter products that may have an impact on heart disease. They can interact with prescription meds, so be sure to discuss them with your doctor.

STEROLS

Sterols are plant fats that are similar in structure to the animal fat cholesterol, except they have a beneficial effect. After you have eaten and digested a sterol, it enters your intestine. In the intestine, it seems to block the absorption of cholesterol across the intestine by blocking the receptors.

Sterols also seem to lower the amount of cholesterol your liver produces in a way not fully understood. Sterols can lower your cholesterol by almost 10 percent if you eat two tablespoons of sterol-containing margarine a day.

B VITAMINS

A high homocysteine level predicts a higher risk of heart disease. Could lowering homocysteine make a difference? A new Swiss heart study says yes. Researchers took patients at high risk for heart disease who had undergone balloon therapy. These patients received a daily vitamin cocktail consisting of folic acid, vitamin B_{12}, and vitamin B_6. After one year, they had a 32 percent decreased risk of heart attack or death (only six months of therapy was necessary to show decreased risk). This decreased risk was over and above the benefit achieved with the balloon therapy.

However, the jury is still out. Two more recent studies showed increased restenosis (narrowing of arteries) or no benefit.

These are the daily dosages used in the Swiss study:

- Folic acid: 1 mg
- Vitamin B_{12}: 400 mg
- Vitamin B_6: 10 mg

COENZYME Q

Coenzyme Q has been widely touted for heart disease. According to Dr. Steven Nissen, "What's legitimate is that it actually may help to prevent the muscle pain that people get on statin drugs."

ANTIOXIDANTS

A study published in *Arteriosclerosis, Thrombosis, and Vascular Biology* suggests that antioxidants (vitamin E, vitamin C, beta-carotene, and selenium) may blunt the effect of cholesterol-lowering drugs. The study showed that drug therapy failed to raise HDL when given with antioxidants. The exact same therapy did raise HDL when antioxidants were not given.

On the other hand, there is a powerful theory that antioxidants may prevent the buildup of plaque. Since, however, the patients in this study already had substantial disease, it is not known if taking supplements earlier in the process might be helpful when medications were not being taken. There are other antioxidant studies ongoing. However, the likelihood of finding major benefit seems low: In the HOPE trial, half the patients also received vitamin E, and no benefit was seen. In earlier clinical trials involving more than 35,000 patients, beta-carotene was compared with placebo and showed no benefit, says Dr. Jeffrey Borer. Dr. Steven Nissen is even more blunt: "Vitamin E doesn't work and may *increase* heart disease."

Vitamin E has long been held as one of the stalwarts of heart disease prevention. However, there is no consensus.

A study of 90,000 nurses suggested that the incidence of heart disease was 30 to 40 percent lower among those with the highest intake of vitamin E from diet and supplements.

In 1994, a study of 5,133 Finnish men and women ages thirty to sixty-nine suggested that increased intake of vitamin E was associated with decreased death from heart disease.

The HOPE trial, the best study looking at the therapeutic benefits of patients given vitamin E to prevent heart disease, failed to find a benefit. The trial studied almost 10,000 patients for four and a half years who were at high risk for heart attack. Those who took 265 mg (400 IU) of vitamin E daily did not experience significantly fewer cardiovascular events or hospitalizations for heart failure or chest pain when compared to those who received a sugar pill. The researchers suggested that it is unlikely that the vitamin E supplement provided any protection against heart disease. This study is continuing to determine whether a longer duration of vitamin E supplements would provide any protection against coronary artery disease.

There are at least two other negative trials with vitamin E. However, Dr. Steven Nissen worries that vitamin E may actually lower HDL levels, doing more damage than good.

ALCOHOL

"Charlie, you don't look so good," I said to Charlie Henneken, at that time a professor of preventive medicine at Harvard Medical School. This was just before the cameras began rolling for a *Dateline NBC* piece.

"Well, I'm not feeling all that well."

"Why?" I asked.

He said, "I've started drinking."

"Why?"

"Well, I've read the literature on drinking and heart disease. I have a strong risk for heart disease and I thought it was a wise preventive measure."

The largest-ever study drives home Charlie's point. Drinking does reduce the risk of heart disease. A twelve-year epidemiological study (unlike a clinical trial, a study without randomized assignment of treatment) of 38,077 male health professionals found that men who drank alcohol three days a week dropped their risk of heart attack by about a third. You've undoubtedly heard about all the benefits of red wine. What sets this study apart is that it's not the kind or quantity that counts so much as the regularity of consumption. Just a half a glass of wine will do. There's no additional benefit to drinking more than two drinks a day. Those who drank five to seven days a week had a slightly lower risk.

The big problem doctors have with recommending drinking as a way to prevent a heart attack is that people have a problem limiting their consumption. In France, where alcohol consumption is high, the rate of heart disease is far lower than in the United States, but many more patients die of cirrhosis of the liver. For that reason, no doctor in his or her right mind would advise you to start drinking to prevent a heart attack, especially since there are so many medications with a much lower risk. However, if you already drink without ill effects, can limit your intake, and are not at risk of alcoholism, alcohol can help prevent heart disease.

The recommended amounts are a 12-ounce bottle of beer, 5 ounces of wine, or 1.5 ounces of 80-proof distilled spirits. Researchers find little difference in effectiveness among these different alcoholic beverages.

HORMONE REPLACEMENT THERAPY

For three decades, doctors promoted HRT as a way of decreasing the risk of heart disease by as much as 50 percent. Now, a study of otherwise healthy women shows a 29 percent *increase* in heart attacks and deaths and a 41 percent *increase* in stroke. This cardiovascular risk, along with a 26 percent increased risk of breast cancer, has made many doctors reconsider the use of HRT.

Who should take HRT? The short answer is probably no one who is not taking it already. In some women, menopausal symptoms are temporary, and HRT was prescribed for short-term use. However, the new research shows an increased risk of heart disease even in the first year of HRT use. So unless your symptoms are constant and debilitating, HRT could be too much of a risk.

If you are already taking HRT, do not discontinue it without consulting your physician. There are newer medications, such as raloxifene (Evista), that decrease the risk of osteoporosis, may decrease the risk of breast cancer, and may lower the risk of heart disease. These do not offer symptom relief, but they do look promising for preventing other effects of menopause. New drugs customized to hit just the right estrogen receptors are in the pipeline.

NUTRITION

Lifestyle changes can add a big punch to your therapy. Reducing saturated fat and cholesterol in your diet, eating plenty of fiber-rich foods, stepping up physical activity, and weight control are the cornerstones of lowering cholesterol. Together they can reduce LDL by 20 to 30 percent, says Dr. James Cleeman, coordinator of the National Cholesterol Education Program of the NHLBI. As you've seen, doubling your drug dose of statins results in only a further 7 percent decrease. As powerful as medications are, the surest way of getting your cholesterol down into a region where you are pulling cholesterol out of your arteries is to add these lifestyle changes to your medications.

Certain foods boost the production of cholesterol in your liver, the powerhouse factory for cholesterol production. Many heart patients try hard to avoid eating cholesterol, not knowing that it's saturated fats, usually animal or dairy fats, that are the biggest villains, spurring the production of cholesterol. Almost as bad are trans fats, which you find in many packaged foods. I was horrified to find these trans-fatty acids on every package of snack food in our local market when I went shopping with my ten-year-old son. Trans fats are just as dangerous as saturated fats yet they are not labeled prominently on packaging. You need to read well down the list of ingredients to see the code words "hydrogenated" or "partially hydrogenated" oils.

Don't assume that other fats are safe. The unsaturated fats found in vegetable oils are still fattening, and obesity adds to the risk of heart disease. The only heart-healthy fats are the omega 3 fats found in fish oil. Even then, all you need are two tablespoons a day. Dr. Steven Nissen summarizes, "Basically statins have the best data. The only reason you don't use a statin is if a patient can't tolerate it, or if a statin alone is not enough. But literally, no one should ever get another agent as the first drug unless he or she can't tolerate a statin. If you're going to do anything, you ought to use the drugs that have this incredible record of reduction in morbidity and mortality."

There is a move afoot to make statins an over-the-counter medication. I personally feel that this is safer than having people take aspirin on their own and may lead to a much better outcome. Once people get a sense of how any amount of statin can start to lower risk, toughen the capsule of vulnerable plaques, I think the enthusiasm will grow for "popping a statin a day." The smart move is still to take enough to lower your LDL well below 100 if you are not at risk for side effects.

Diet is a huge issue in heart disease. Token efforts were made by many patients in the past to lower their cholesterol simply by cutting down on animal fats in their diet. Now those efforts have become even weaker for millions of Americans because of the amazing efficacy of statins. However, a new study in *JAMA* shows that a rigorous diet can be just as powerful as statins in reducing cholesterol levels. Many patients don't put in the effort. However, if you are dedicated, diets like Dean Ornish's have been documented to work well, actually reversing the blockages found in coronary arteries. Increasingly, heart disease is seen as a lifestyle disease. I personally rely on a very rigorous exercise program and diet to keep my cholesterol in check. "Clearly the consumer has to understand that this disease begins silently at an early age," says Dr. Lewis Kuller of the University of Pittsburgh. "Young people have to be made aware of the fact that they've got to keep their LDL cholesterol down and that's mainly not drug therapy. It's diet and lifestyle modification." And remember, metabolic syndrome is *entirely* a lifestyle disease.

Although this chapter is very heavily oriented toward drugs, the proof is that exercise, lifestyle changes, and nutrition for the disciplined can be just as effective—these are the measures I personally take and advocate.

EXERCISE

Regular exercise is clearly correlated with decreased rate of death, fewer heart attacks, and greater longevity. The best epidemiological studies show that it is the quantity, not intensity, of exercise that improves health. "You don't need to run a 10-K, but you ought to get in roughly half an hour of exercise a day," says Dr. Sidney Smith, past president of the American Heart Association. "There are all types of opportunities in daily life where we can get exercise. I happen to run in the morning, but I also, in the midst of my life, look for ways to get activity. Swimming, cycling, rowing are all activities that don't hammer away at the knees and build up good endurance."

Exercise is even more important for women than men. A recent study in *Circulation* showed that for every 1 MET increase in exercise capacity, there was a 17 percent decrease in death. A MET is a measure of exercise found by defining the amount of oxygen used by the average person at rest. Two METs is roughly equivalent to walking less than 2 mph, 5 METs is roughly walking at 4 mph, and 8 METs is jogging at 6 mph.

However, if you are at high risk and can't meet your goal with diet and exercise changes, then you need to consider drug therapy.

Throughout this book I've looked at how half of Americans with heart disease die suddenly and without apparent warning. From this chapter, you can see that among the missing half are those who don't take the right medications or who don't take them in the right amounts or for a long enough time to be effective. Add to that those who simply take a single cholesterol- or blood-pressure-lowering drug without achieving their goals.

The right medications play a huge role in preventing heart

attacks and premature death. The earlier you are on the right medications, the less chance of your ever needing surgery. Remember, this is a progressive disease. If you can slow, stop, or even reverse this progression, you'll live far better-quality years and far more years. Although any one measure can decrease your risk by as much as 38 percent, combining these measures can decrease your risk by 60 percent.

STEP SEVEN: GET THE RIGHT LIFESAVING PROCEDURE

Fatal Flaw

"Have you seen a priest?" The words put the fear of God into the man lying on an ambulance stretcher in the arrivals area of the hospital's emergency department. I could hardly believe that a senior cardiologist would have so little tact in introducing himself to the patient who was writhing in pain. He had a type 1 dissecting aortic aneurysm, which was beginning to close off his coronary arteries. There is a lifesaving technique for this heart condition. Unfortunately, the hospital had performed few of them and the cardiac surgeon on call had done even fewer.

Hours later, the patient died a sudden, agonizing, and convulsive death. He had been referred to this hospital center by his family doctor, but it was the wrong one. For any major heart procedure, the best predictor of a favorable outcome is volume. If the key to good real estate is location, location, location, the key to great hospital care is volume, volume, volume. Unfortunately, this hospital's volume of patients with aneurysms was near zero. The lack of experience doomed the patient.

Conventional wisdom: *My doctor right or wrong.*
The real deal: *Better be sure he or she's not dead wrong.*

Choosing a hospital that does too few procedures to be good is just one of the mistakes consumers make in pursuing the best care. Here are the other common errors:

- Failing to look at the hospital's scorecard for excellent results
- Failing to determine if the procedure is appropriate for you
- Failing to determine if the right procedure has been selected for your needs
- Failing to choose an excellent physician or surgeon with proven results

This chapter will help you avoid these common mistakes and become a terrific health care consumer.

"Techniques for performing heart procedures have improved so dramatically over the last fifteen years that the risk of performing these procedures has been minimized and the benefits that you can expect after successful performance of them have increased considerably," says Dr. Jeffrey Borer.

The other big change is that even patients who are sicker still do extremely well. Dr. Steven Nissen says, "The average patient undergoing open-heart surgery today is many years older than he or she was even a decade ago. We're not seeing patients in their fifties; we're seeing them in their sixties, seventies, and older. We even bypass people in their eighties and, occasionally, I've even sent patients close to ninety years old. And so the risks have remained constant primarily because the patients' age and the co-morbidities have gotten worse and worse while the surgery has improved. But if you're a sixty-year-old man having his first bypass operation, your risk is minuscule."

Medications are also making a big difference in terms of safety and recovery. "There have been huge advances with safety," says Dr. Nissen. "For instance, the potent intravenous anti-platelet agents are really extraordinarily effective at lowering the risk of heart attack and other serious complications during interventional therapy."

The first key issue is whether the procedure is right for your condition. As many as 25 percent of medical procedures and surgeries are considered inappropriate. (With the scrutiny applied to bypass surgery, that number is likely to be lower.) If yours is inappropriate, avoiding the procedure can save you from the risk of complications or death. Here's an example told to me by an eminent surgeon.

A man in his fifties had a balloon therapy, which was not clearly appropriate. Afterward, the artery was scarred from the procedure. The man then required bypass surgery since the artery had narrowed, or "stenosed." To make it more palatable he was offered a new off-bypass technique (surgery without use of the heart-lung machine). Surgeons also convinced him that it was urgent, that he couldn't go to any other hospital or get a second opinion.

Surgeons attempted to do an off-bypass procedure through a small "keyhole" (so-called minimally invasive surgery). With the restricted visibility of the procedure, surgeons accidentally made a hole in the right ventricle. In an oh-my-God-don't-let-him-die move, surgeons now had to crash—put the patient on bypass and rip open his chest. Surgeons fixed the hole, but only after transfusing between twenty and thirty units of blood and the patient's blood pressure dropping to a perilously low level.

After the surgery, he had complications, lots of them, including high fevers. Surgeons now considered another course, robotic surgery. They decided against it because, as an experimental procedure that currently requires more time than conventional surgery and leaves the surgeon with less direct control of the structures in the chest than conventional surgery, it seemed an imprudent choice.

Finally, he went to another hospital where, to their horror, doctors found that he had a major infection in his sternum plus pus in his chest. He required more surgery for treatment of the infection and a long hospitalization.

Two years later he still has chest pain, and tests show that the bypass grafts have considerably narrowed. Now when he tries to walk or jog more than a block, his muscles tighten up and he has excruciating pain.

Horror stories like this one are not reflected in the statistics. The lesson is simple: Make sure you really need a procedure and be certain that the procedure you decide on is appropriate and will be performed by the right surgeons in a hospital with vast experience with your problem.

Now let's look at how to get the best possible outcome with the lowest risk if the procedure is necessary and appropriate. The two key therapies are balloon therapy and coronary artery bypass surgery. In all of consumer medicine, treatment of coronary artery disease is the most advanced. There are a few solid criteria you can apply to selecting the correct procedure that are simpler and easier to use than those for buying a car. The same is true for vascular surgery.

In considering the choice between these two procedures, you are dealing with natural competition between surgeons and cardiologists for patients. In the following pages you will encounter some very forceful and convincing doctors who argue strongly for their position. I do not take a position that one procedure is superior to the other. There is an even more forceful argument that very aggressive drug therapy may so radically reduce risk that the number of these procedures in the future could be dramatically reduced. In researching this book, I found outright anger in each camp at the views of other. I've spared you the drama, but keep in mind that each faction tightly holds its own view.

BALLOON THERAPY AND STENTING

Balloon therapy, technically termed angioplasty, made its debut in 1977 as the biggest revolution in cardiology since bypass surgery. The concept was simple: Position a small balloon into the center of a narrowed artery, open the balloon, and widen the artery. Although it seemed very simple, the first procedure was fraught with danger. "It was extremely dangerous to dilate the arteries of patients suffering from sudden chest pain or a heart attack," says Dr. Jeffrey Moses. What's changed? "The catheters onto which the balloons are fit are infinitely better. What's more, in the 1970s, 40 percent returned within three years because the artery narrowed again. Over the decades this has improved dramatically so that it can be performed as an outpatient procedure." For practical purposes, as you'll see, balloon therapy has been largely enhanced with what is termed stenting.

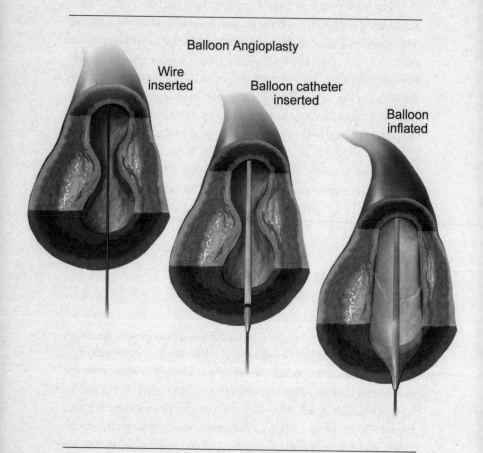

Balloon Angioplasty

Wire
inserted

Balloon catheter
inserted

Balloon
inflated

HOW THE PROCEDURE IS DONE

Your cardiologist makes a small incision in your groin under local anesthesia, then threads a long, thin, hollow tube up through the aorta and into the artery in your heart that is partially blocked. Near the end of the tube is a balloon. Once that balloon is centered in your artery within the area of the partial blockage, your cardiologist inflates the balloon, hoping to push the blockage aside. That seems simple enough. The problem is that the blockage could re-form, or pieces of it could even break loose.

That's why it's now common practice for the cardiologist to place a pipelike device called a stent into the artery to prop it open. Even with a stent, 20 percent of patients still require another balloon procedure within a year to reopen the blood vessel. According to New York State statistics, 37 percent of stents fail after four years. Cardiologist Steven Nissen disagrees that the failure rate is so high.

Stenosis is the narrowing of a blood vessel. Restenosis can occur when scar tissue forms in or around the site where the stent was placed. To prevent restenosis, manufacturers have invented new drug-coated stents, called drug-eluting stents. These are narrow mesh tubes coated with a medication that acts to prevent the scarring in an artery that can cause it to narrow and "reclog."

Currently in the United States, more than 1 million stents are placed in patients annually during angioplasty procedures. Anytime a balloon is used in a coronary artery, the lining of the artery is damaged and is prone to scarring, which can close it down again. Let's take a look at one of the most promising stents made by Johnson and Johnson. (A second drug-eluting stent, made by Boston Scientific, is entering the U.S. market.) Half a million have already been implanted.

CYPHER STENT

The Cypher stent contains an immunosuppressive drug, sirolimus, to prevent restenosis. Dr. Jeffrey Moses was the lead investigator in the SIRIUS study, which resulted in the FDA approval of Cypher. The study results showed that 90 percent of the patients had no scarring with the drug-coated stents, as opposed to 70 percent of patients being scar-free with uncoated stents. Dr. Moses believes it will revolutionize the field of interventional cardiology. Other studies have shown that the restenosis risk has been cut to less than 5 percent with the new drug-coated stents. Even though these stents will likely become the standard of care during balloon therapy, their long-term benefits and risks still remain unknown. Long-term animal studies suggest that restenosis may still occur years later. Dr. Moses counters that animals are not good models for humans and that in four years of follow-up, "We're reasonably confident that there's not much creep."

There is one long-term study, led by Dr. J. Eduardo Sousa of the Institute Dante Pazzanese of Cardiology in São Paulo. Researchers from Brazil, Florida, the Netherlands, and Boston, evaluated the clinical outcomes of patients who received the sirolimus-eluting stents two years earlier. They used an incredibly sophisticated technique—placing an ultrasound device into the coronary artery to look at changes in the stent. Half of the patients in the study had received the slow-release stent and half had received the fast-release stent. Twenty-eight patients were available for the follow-up. None of the patients suffered in-stent restenosis. One patient in the fast-release group required revascularization. They found that in-stent regrowth was minimal. Only three patients in the entire group required revascularization.

The researchers concluded from their small study that the stents remain safe and effective for forty-eight months after implantation, although there was slightly more narrowing in the fast-release group. Currently about 95 percent of balloon therapy patients receive stents. Those who don't often have vessels too small to accommodate a stent.

Dr. Wayne Isom is still cautious: "Unless you see five years of results, all of this stuff is pure speculation. All those studies have a small number of patients. You can kind of summarize it in that the early results sound good with the drug-eluting stents, but we're going to have to wait three to four more years." Dr. Jeffrey Moses counters that many experts think the drug-coated stents are going to surpass bypass surgery. "Surgery is declining. In the last couple of years in the United States, it's down 20 percent. It's because we're replacing it. The drug-eluting stents haven't even hit yet and it's still declining. The interventional therapy [angioplasty] with its newfound durability is going to dominate. There's no question about it."

The key consumer point is be certain you are getting the most up-to-date stent technology. As of now, the sirolimus is among the best. The higher your risk of restenosis, the more you should consider one. Be certain also that before your procedure begins, doctors have the right size stents for your arteries.

Some patients have ended up with a mix of old and new stents in their arteries, which leaves them with the restenosis rate of the old stent.

There was another controversy. In July 2003 and again in October 2003, the Food and Drug Administration issued safety notices to doctors linking Cypher to blood clots that formed within thirty days after patients had received the new device. The agency noted a number of deaths but said that it did not have enough information to determine whether those deaths could be attributed to the new stent procedure. In issuing these safety notices, the FDA said it had received more than 290 reports of blood clots among Cypher recipients, more than 60 of which led to patient deaths.

The agency, which monitors the situation daily, has also received more than 50 reports of allergic-type reactions among Cypher stent recipients. Trials showed about a 3 percent allergy rate among recipients of both Cypher and bare stents. But blaming the stent can be difficult because heart patients take many drugs.

The FDA said it did not know the cause of the problems and did not yet have enough data to determine whether the Cypher stent was riskier than the bare metal stent. Dr. Jeffrey Moses counters, "The FDA has subsequently acknowledged that there is no difference between these and regular stents. There is no specific problem. That, of course, didn't make the headlines. The allergies were from the ancillary meds. There are no issues with those either."

As this book goes to press, Boston Scientific, manufacturer of the Taxus drug-coated stent, has recalled these stents after three deaths and several injuries. Initial reports indicate that the balloon did not deflate properly at the end of the procedure. Your cardiologist will be able to tell you if this problem has been eliminated.

CONSUMER QUESTION #1: SHOULD YOU CONSIDER BALLOON THERAPY?

Here are the key indications for balloon therapy.

Symptom relief. The primary indication for balloon therapy is to relieve persistent chest pain that is not controllable by medication or lifestyle changes. There is still no conclusive evidence that balloon therapy prolongs life for most people with coronary disease. So although the procedure may fix your pain, it may not save your life when used for chronic stable chest pain.

Your coronary arteries may be lined with dozens of highly toxic plaques, all vulnerable to fracture. The angiogram may find one or two that protrude into your arteries and are highly visible. Balloon therapy effectively removes those blockages but leaves behind dozens of potentially deadly "submerged" plaques. Over the next year, one of those can fracture and cause a heart attack. Angioplasty does not get at the basic disease process. Only intensive medical therapy can change the course of the disease.

EXPERT COUNSEL
Dr. Thomas Graboys: "My message to patients is if you have no symptoms and are feeling well, the risk of proceeding to a catheterization and a stent may well be greater than the benefit. And there is no evidence that putting all these stents in prolongs people's lives except for the small group who are unstable."

During a heart attack. If you're having a heart attack, balloon therapy can save your life and prevent a great deal of damage to your heart. Balloon therapy stops the heart attack and does so faster than bypass surgery. Dr. Wayne Isom says, "One of the reasons that angioplasty has got better results is you can get patients to the cath lab, get everything prepared, and get that thing open quicker than you can bypass surgery."

How much better is balloon therapy than clot-busting drugs? Here are two expert opinions.

Angioplasty and stents are a much better solution for treating a heart attack, cutting deaths by 40–50 percent above and beyond those of clot busters. That's saying a lot. (Remember that clot busters dissolve the clot in a coronary artery to restore blood flow.) Says Dr. Jeffrey Moses, "We know with heart attacks, the best therapy you can have is angioplasty. It saves lives over clot busters."

Dr. Jeffrey Borer notes that angioplasty offers a 1–2 percent mortality reduction compared with clot busters; this may be a relative risk reduction of as much as 20 percent, which is why it is preferable to do an angioplasty if possible. But clotbusters remain a very effective treatment, especially if angioplasty is not immediately available. "I think, however, that the 40 to 50 percent reduction in relative risk may come from the most optimistic comparisons," says Dr. Borer.

Bottom line: If you're having a heart attack and can't get to a great institution that performs angioplasty, consider clot-busting drugs.

Unstable angina. This is new, worsening chest pain but still not classified as a heart attack because heart muscle is not being destroyed. Dr. Jeffrey Moses says, "Unstable angina is referred to as a near miss heart attack, where many of the signs and symptoms are present but it doesn't complete itself and damage the heart muscle. These patients do much better if they have an angioplasty with a stent than if they just get medical therapy."

Shock. A recent study examined patients already in shock. They used to die despite heroic efforts. Their hearts didn't beat strongly enough to support their internal organs even at rest; tissue throughout the body began to die; they had extremely low blood pressure, were cold, clammy, and confused, and their kidneys were failing. A recent study published in the *New England Journal of Medicine* showed that angioplasty or bypass surgery does not significantly reduce deaths of shock patients at thirty days (the primary end point of the study); however, after six months, patients who had these procedures performed early had a 35 percent improvement in survival over patients who received intensive drug therapy, including clot busters. The improvement in survival was even greater (57 percent) for patients under seventy-five years. "These results provide evidence that early treatment with bypass surgery or angioplasty can save the lives of heart attack patients with cardiogenic shock. Physicians should be strongly encouraged to consider emergency revascularization for these patients, even if it means referring them to another hospital that is better equipped to handle these procedures," says Dr. Claude Lenfant.

Each year, 71,000 patients with heart attacks develop shock while in the hospital. The key action point is to act early at the very first signs of shock, to be certain you are in a hospital capable of performing balloon therapy under adverse conditions.

Abnormal angiogram. The angiogram is the gold standard test for locating and planning treatment of blockages in coronary arteries. This critical test allows your doctors to decide which is best for you: balloon therapy, bypass surgery, or medical therapy. The following results might point you toward balloon therapy and stenting.

- Major blockage of any single coronary artery, which is not a major artery. "Just about everyone agrees that unless you have got at least 50 to 60 percent blockage it's not a significant blockage," says Dr. Wayne Isom. Significant blockages have three categories: Mild is 50–65 percent; moderate is 65–80 percent; severe is 80–90 percent. Dr. Jeffrey Borer argues that "angioplasty for patients with single-vessel disease is justified only for symptom relief or if the asymptomatic but objectively ischemic patient wants to undertake a very active lifestyle without lifestyle-limiting medications. There is no clear basis for angioplasty for single-vessel disease just because it is there and, certainly, no evidence that MI or death is prevented."
- The left anterior descending. Dr. Jeffrey Moses's group at Lenox Hill performs balloon therapy on some left main coronary arteries. Some other doctors consider balloon

therapy too risky in these patients because their heart might shut down; they prefer to do a bypass. During bypass surgery, the patient is on a heart-lung machine until the heart is ready to beat on its own.

- Major blockage of up to three arteries if your heart has normal pump function. Again, the left main coronary artery is excluded. Many surgeons argue that with three blockages, you should consider bypass surgery. With so many stents, if these vessels reocclude, it will be very hard later to find a place to bypass a vessel. Also, there are no data showing that you will live longer with balloon therapy. Nevertheless, many skilled cardiologists feel comfortable with multiple-vessel balloon procedures.

- Major blockage of any two arteries if you have only moderate pump function. Dr. Jeffrey Borer notes that angioplasty is a reasonable therapy here, for example, in someone whose test results show a severe lack of blood flow to the heart muscle. He adds, though, that "even this might be debated."

Other conditions. Here's a brief list of other conditions where balloon therapy is indicated.

- Chest pain continues after a heart attack. Bypass surgery should be considered as well, depending on the number of vessels that are narrowed and their locations.

- Cardiac arrest that can't be linked to a heart attack. If, however, you have diffuse disease and poor function of your left ventricle, your doctor may consider an implantable defibrillator instead.

- Before major surgery if you have chest pain or poor blood flow to parts of your heart. A common example is joint replacement surgery, which can place a major strain on your heart. Your surgeon often obtains a workup of your heart's health before surgery. It's during that workup that cardiac problems may be found that would pose a significant risk during surgery if not corrected.

- If you're athletic and have chest pain when you exercise that cannot be treated with medication.
- When you cannot tolerate the side effects of medications that are necessary to treat your chest pain.
- If you have a very abnormal stress test even without symptoms.

CONSUMER QUESTION #2: IS BALLOON THERAPY INAPPROPRIATE IN YOUR CASE?

Some surgeons believe that too many angioplasties are performed. In 2001 in New York State, there were 42,000 angioplasties and only 16,000 bypass surgeries.

You may want to attribute part of this to the natural competition between cardiologists and surgeons. With advances in techniques, skill, catheters, and stents, cardiologists are taking away more and more of the surgeons' business. Still, you should be aware of cases where angioplasty is clearly not appropriate.

Here are some situations when angioplasty should not be performed.

- You haven't given medication a fair trial. Thousands of balloon therapies are performed each year on patients who push their doctors into acting too quickly. It can take weeks and even months to experience the full effect of many drugs.
- Multiple angioplasties must be performed over time and your cardiac function may deteriorate as a result. Dr. Wayne Isom counsels that "if it doesn't work the first

time, get another opinion before you continue repeated angioplasties."

- Your angiogram shows extensive, severe blockages.
- No emergency surgical backup is available if your balloon therapy fails and you require bypass surgery.
- You have diabetes. In 1995, the NHLBI issued a clinical alert to U.S. physicians on results from the BARI study. It found that patients with diabetes who were treated with bypass surgery had a markedly lower death rate after five years than similar patients treated with angioplasty. Cardiologist Steven Nissen says the BARI data are very clear and he doesn't see the case for angioplasty in diabetics. Diabetics may have better long-term outcomes with the new drug-eluting stents, counters Dr. Jeffrey Moses. "The real restenosis rate is in the teens. But it's still not settled in multivessel diabetics which way we should go with them."

RISKS

Balloon therapy appears incredibly simple, and the number of patients who do very well is large. Yet there are still real dangers and you should be aware of them and of your individual risk for them. Among the most serious are

- Postangioplasty hemorrhage with anemia
- Intermediate coronary syndrome
- Acute lung edema
- Respiratory failure
- Acute kidney failure
- Shock
- Accidental laceration
- Heart attack

Review your risk of these with your cardiologist. Here are some expert opinions to consider.

EXPERT COUNSEL
Dr. Jeffrey Borer says, "There is still indeed the possibility of unnecessary balloon therapy, if by unnecessary we mean that it was meant to prolong someone's life. There are no data that suggest you would prolong someone's life. All the big studies with angioplasty have shown that heart attack rate postangioplasty remains relatively high."

EXPERT COUNSEL
Dr. Steven Nissen has a reasonable explanation for this. "Underneath the plaques when you perform an angioplasty, there are still substances that can cause blood to clot. It's a reasonably credible explanation for why heart attacks are so frequent."

Unless your condition is immediately life-threatening, take the time to get a second (and even third) opinion—if only to reassure yourself that you are making the right decision. Dr. Wayne Isom stresses that "most good cardiologists and cardiac surgeons are going to agree 90 percent of the time on how the patient should be treated. Even people like myself, Moses, Borer—in most instances we'd agree which way a patient should be treated. It's not that big a debate."

CONSUMER QUESTION #3: WHAT'S YOUR CHANCE OF SUCCESS?

Before you decide on angioplasty, you should ask your doctors to grade your chance of success based on the severity of the blockage. Blockages are graded A, B, and C. A blockages are like driving down a wide-open eight-lane highway. C blockages are like small, tortuous mountain goatpaths. B blockages are somewhere in between. Your cardiologist will review the findings on your angiogram to determine which blockage you may have.

TYPE A BLOCKAGE

Balloon therapy performed on type A blockages has a high success rate (more than 90 percent). In competent hands, these should be easy to operate on. They have all of the following characteristics.

- Discrete blockage that is less than 10 mm in length
- Concentric (ringing the artery wall)
- Smooth contour
- Little or no calcification, indicating that the blockage has not been present long enough to harden
- Readily accessible
- Not at a sharp turn in the artery (less than 45 degrees)
- Artery less than totally blocked
- No significant involvement of a major artery branch
- No blood clot

TYPE B BLOCKAGE

Type B blockages have a medium success rate (85–90 percent) with balloon therapy. In expert hands, you can still have a good outcome due to better techniques, better equipment, and more experience. They have the following characteristics.

- Tubular, 10–20 mm long
- Eccentric (concentrated on one side of the artery)

- Irregular contour
- Moderate to heavy calcification
- Moderate tortuosity of first part of the artery (twists and turns are present that can make maneuvering the catheter difficult)
- Located at a moderate turn in the artery (greater than 45 degrees but less than 90 degrees), at the opening of an artery, or at the point where an artery divides
- Total occlusions that are less than three months old (regular angiograms must be taken for this to be known)
- Some blood clot present

TYPE C BLOCKAGE

Balloon therapy has only a 60–70 percent success rate with type C blockages. The following characteristics may cause you to abandon balloon therapy or consider bypass surgery.

- Degenerated vein grafts from previous bypass surgery or very rough contours
- Total occlusion more than three months old, as seen on angiograms (the blockage is older and harder)
- Excessive tortuosity of first part of artery (too many twists and turns for the catheter to maneuver well)
- A sharp (90-degree) turn in the artery (maneuvering the catheter becomes as difficult as threading a twisted coat hanger through a straw)
- Inability to protect major side branches of the artery (which could shut down, thereby stopping the flow of blood to the heart if the procedure is unsuccessful)

The most important criterion for success is how healthy your heart muscle itself is before the procedure. Dr. Jeffrey

Moses counters that this does not mean that bypass surgery is the better treatment for patients with weaker hearts.

Patients with substantial disease in all three main coronary arteries, or with diabetes, are better candidates for surgery than they are for balloon therapy, say cardiac surgeons. Surgeons can't operate on patients with two or three steel stents in an artery (they call this "the full metal jacket"). There is no place left to connect the bypass graft. Bottom line, look at the long view. Are you going to need multiple balloon procedures over time? If so, consider your odds with surgery. Surgery has the advantage of one-stop shopping. Consider these data from New York State. Patients with balloon therapy had a 40 percent chance of returning for more balloon therapy or even bypass surgery within four years. (Most reoccurrence was between six and eighteen months.) With stents, the return rate is markedly reduced, and with drug-eluting stents even more drastically reduced, adds Dr. Jeffrey Moses.

With surgery, however, the chance of coming back for more surgery in four years was just 1 percent, claim surgeons. The need for angioplasty in the first year after surgery is 3 percent, according to Dr. Jeffrey Moses, citing the ARTS, ERACI II, and SOS trials. So if you want to be done with it, surgery can be a better choice. These data do come from the pre-stent days, so cardiologists are eagerly awaiting new data as they are reported.

Listen to two other experts who also have reservations about angioplasty.

EXPERT COUNSEL
Dr. Lewis Kuller: "I think there are too many angioplasties done because I think basically this is a systemic disease. And the only people who really need angioplasty are those who are symptomatic. I think it's just done because there is so much disease out there. Basically all

men have severe disease when they get into the older age groups. If someone walks in and says he doesn't feel so hot, and you send him for an angiogram, the chances are pretty high that you are going to find disease that you think requires an angioplasty. That's a paradigm that's hard to change."

EXPERT COUNSEL

Dr. Jeffrey Borer: "Personally, when I see people who have prognostically severe coronary disease, that is, severe multivessel disease with high-grade ischemia [reduction in blood flow], I send them to surgery. I don't try to do multivessel angioplasties. On the other hand, I'm very happy to have angioplasties performed on patients who are unhappy with the side effects of drugs."

WOMEN

It used to be the case that women did not do nearly as well as men with either balloon therapy or bypass surgery. They were diagnosed late, so were by then sicker, and they have smaller, harder to operate on blood vessels. Now, in a major triumph, the NHLBI reveals that women undergoing coronary artery bypass surgery or balloon angioplasty procedures to improve blood flow to the heart survive just as well as men. Five years after receiving bypass or angioplasty, 87 percent of women enrolled in the Bypass Angioplasty Revascularization Investigation (BARI) had survived, compared to men's 88 percent survival rate. Women in the BARI study were older than the men, and had more congestive heart failure, diabetes, high blood pressure, and high blood cholesterol—and still they did just as well. Unfortunately, many women still do not get adequate medical

treatment, failing to have many lifesaving medications prescribed for them, which is why they are much sicker when they
finally get to surgery. My own mother was allowed to collapse
in fulminant congestive heart failure before surgery was performed.

CONSUMER QUESTION #4:
DO YOU HAVE THE RIGHT
CARDIOLOGIST FOR
BALLOON THERAPY?

Just like rating a baseball player, cardiologists can be rated
based on their outcomes and the number and kind of procedures
they do. For instance, a cardiologist could have terrific scores
operating on A blockages but have little or no experience on Cs.
Also be careful with numbers of cases done. Dr. Jeffrey Borer advises, "Ask him! If he says, 'The team here has done eighty
cases,' well, 'the team'? Does that mean there are ten cardiologists each of whom has done eight procedures? Volume is key."

"You definitely want volume," agrees Dr. Jeffrey Moses.
"You want to go to a center that does a lot. That helps. And you
want a cardiologist to do a lot. The minimal standard is considered seventy-five, but in reality, I promise you, you want to go to
someone who does several hundred a year. I would say a minimum of two hundred a year. I do a thousand. And you want to
know what the complication rates are and the mortality rates.
You want to go to a center that does a thousand or more a year,
certainly at least five hundred. Then the team is there, I promise
you. They're grooved, they're used to it, they handle high volume. Some people think, you do a lot of them, you lose track.
No, the more you do, the better the team gets. A surgeon may do
two hundred, but if his center does only two hundred, that's not
so great. Basically, you want a guy who does two hundred in a
center that does at least five hundred."

CONSUMER QUESTION #5: HOW DO YOU PICK THE RIGHT HOSPITAL?

It may surprise you to learn that choosing an excellent hospital is simpler than picking a car based on consumer report ratings. The hard work of accumulating masses of data and analyzing them has been done. HealthGrades, Inc. has graciously allowed me to reprint their list of top five-star hospitals.

Although there are many different criteria you could apply, excellent results are the hallmark of the best centers. Health-Grades purchased the initial data from the Centers for Medicare and Medicaid (CMS), then analyzed patient outcome data for virtually every hospital in the country. The Medicare data (MedPAR file) from CMS contained the inpatient records for Medicare patients. Hospitals were required by law to submit complete and accurate information with substantial penalties for reporting inaccurate or incomplete data. The Medicare population has another advantage—it represents a majority of the patients for all of the clinical categories studied, with approximately 60 percent of all cardiac patients.

Risk factors were analyzed, as were postsurgical complications. A top academic center like Mass General in Boston accepts very difficult cases with great technical complexity in very sick patients and this could lower their score. HealthGrades took this into consideration and also weighed risks including age, sex, specific procedure performed, and coexisting conditions such as hypertension, chronic renal failure, congestive heart failure, and diabetes.

Some surgeons perform so well that even with an incredibly complex patient mix, they—and their hospitals—still get great results. Wayne Isom at New York–Presbyterian, Weill Cornell Medical Center; Laurence Cohn at the Brigham and Women's Hospital; and Toby Cosgrove at the Cleveland Clinic see some of the most difficult cases in the world.

HealthGrades has three ratings. In five-star hospitals, actual performance was better than predicted and the difference was statistically significant. In three-star hospitals, actual performance was not significantly different from what was predicted. In one-star hospitals, actual performance was worse than predicted and the difference was statistically significant.

Here is HealthGrades's list of five-star hospitals, which scored highest for interventional procedures including PTCA/angioplasty, stent, and atherectomy.

CALIFORNIA
Mt. Diablo Medical Center, Concord
St. Helena Hospital, Deer Park
Scripps Memorial Hospital, Encinitas
Scripps Green Hospital, La Jolla
Good Samaritan Hospital, Los Angeles
Doctors Medical Center, Modesto
Sequoia Hospital, Redwood City
St. John's Hospital Health Center, Santa Monica

CONNECTICUT
Bridgeport Hospital, Bridgeport
Yale New Haven Hospital, New Haven

FLORIDA
Florida Hospital, Orlando
Halifax Medical Center, Daytona Beach
Munroe Regional Medical Center, Ocala
Holy Cross Hospital, Fort Lauderdale
Florida Medical Center, Fort Lauderdale
Sarasota Memorial Hospital, Sarasota
Lawnwood Regional Medical Center, Fort Pierce
Morton Plant Hospital, Clearwater
Holmes Regional Medical Center, Melbourne

Naples Community Hospital, Naples
Palm Beach Gardens Medical Center, Palm Beach Gardens
Regional Medical Center Bayonet Point, Hudson

GEORGIA
Saint Joseph's Hospital, Atlanta

IDAHO
St. Luke's Regional Medical Center, Boise

ILLINOIS
St. John's Hospital, Springfield
Memorial Medical Center, Springfield

IOWA
Mercy Medical Center, Dubuque

INDIANA
St. Vincent Hospital, Indianapolis
Community Hospital, Munster

LOUISIANA
Lafayette General Medical Center, Lafayette
Thibodaux Regional Medical Center, Thibodaux

MAINE
Maine Medical Center, Portland

MARYLAND
Union Memorial Hospital, Baltimore
Washington Adventist Hospital, Baltimore

MASSACHUSETTS
Brigham and Women's Hospital, Boston

MICHIGAN
Munson Medical Center, Traverse City
William Beaumont Hospital, Royal Oak
St. Mary's Medical Center, Saginaw

MINNESOTA
Abbott Northwestern Hospital, Minneapolis

MONTANA
Deaconess Billings Clinic, Billings
St. Patrick Hospital, Missoula

NEVADA
Sunrise Hospital and Medical Center, Las Vegas

NEW HAMPSHIRE
Portsmouth Regional Hospital, Portsmouth

NEW JERSEY
Hackensack University Medical, Hackensack
Newark Beth Israel Medical Center, Newark
Morristown Memorial Hospital, Morristown
Robert Wood Johnson University Hospital, New
     Brunswick

NEW YORK
Buffalo General Hospital–Kaledia Health, Buffalo
Mt. Sinai Hospital, New York City
St. Luke's–Roosevelt Hospital, New York City
Lenox Hill Hospital, New York City
New York Hospital Medical Center of Queens, Flushing
St. Peter's Hospital, Albany
Montefiore Medical Center, Bronx
Westchester Medical Center, Valhalla
North Shore University Hospital, Manhasset

Rochester General Hospital, Rochester
Winthrop University Hospital, Mineola
St. Francis Hospital, Roslyn
Maimondides Medical Center, Brooklyn
Long Island Jewish Medical Center, New Hyde Park
St. Elizabeth's Hospital, Utica
St. Joseph's Hospital Health Center, Syracuse

NORTH CAROLINA
Mercy Hospital, Charlotte

NORTH DAKOTA
St. Alexius Medical Center, Bismarck

OHIO
Southwest General Center, Middleburg Heights
EMH Regional Medical Center, Elyria
Christ Hospital, Cincinnati
St. Elizabeth Health Center, Youngstown

PENNSYLVANIA
Saint Vincent Health System, Erie
Hamot Medical Center, Erie
York Hospital, York
UPMC Shadyside, Pittsburgh
St. Mary Medical Center, Langhorne
Altoona Hospital, Altoona
Lancaster General Hospital, Lancaster
Presbyterian University of Pennsylvania Medical Center,
    Philadelphia

SOUTH DAKOTA
Avera McKennan Hospital and University Health Center,
    Sioux Falls

TENNESSEE
Blount Memorial Hospital, Maryville

TEXAS
Medical Center Hospital, Odessa
Scott and White Memorial Hospital, Temple
Texoma Medical Center, Denison

VIRGINIA
Sentara Norfolk General Hospital, Norfolk

WISCONSIN
Wausau Hospital, Wausau
Bellin Memorial Hospital, Green Bay
St. Luke's Medical Center, Milwaukee

Dr. Jeffrey Moses adds Indianapolis Heart, and Swedish Hospital in Seattle, which are contemporary "hot spots" for angioplasty. In the next five years, Dr. Moses predicts that there will be specialized angioplasty centers: "In the same way that if you're in a car accident on the road, they send you to a major trauma center, with a heart attack or chest pain, you'll be sent to a specialized angioplasty center."

What should you do if you need angioplasty and there is no five-star hospital nearby? If you have the money and time, certainly you should travel to one of the best hospitals. Otherwise, go to the HealthGrades Web site (www.healthgrades.com) and check their list of three-star hospitals near you. Finally, keep in mind that even one-star hospitals perform many more successful than unsuccessful procedures. And their doctors are gaining valuable experience every day. If you must have your angioplasty performed at one of these hospitals, try to get the doctor who has the most experience. I've found five-star doctors at three-star hospitals.

CONSUMER QUESTION #6:
ARE YOU GETTING THE PROPER
POSTPROCEDURE CARE?

The first rule afterward is no smoking—no exceptions, no excuses.

Postprocedure care can make a bigger life-and-death difference than the procedure itself. Post-procedure has two parts: first, medications to help prevent short-term complications; second, medications to treat the underlying disease. Unfortunately, the majority of angioplasty patients are not treated adequately for their underlying disease, says Dr. Steven Nissen. To minimize your chance of a complication after stents, be certain you take these medications long enough to make a difference.

- Cholesterol-lowering therapy. Statins are strongly recommended.
- Ace inhibitors.
- Antiplatelet therapy/blood thinners. The current recommendation is twelve months on aspirin or clot-reducing drugs (up from the previous recommendation of four weeks).

Dr. Jeffrey Moses advises, "If you have coronary disease, you should take aspirin, unless there's an allergy or a real bleeding problem. And it's important that, in general, the chronic dose of aspirin probably should be 81 mg."

Dr. Lewis Kuller adds, "Clopidogrel (Plavix) is more potent than aspirin, and both drugs actually work better when used together. The most important time to give clopidogrel is after angioplasty. In fact, it is considered greatly inappropriate not to give it after angioplasty unless the patient has had a severe allergic reaction to it." Dr. Moses agrees: "Clopidogrel with the stent is really mandatory for thirty days and, with the new drug-eluting stents, at least three months. Here at Lenox Hill, we prescribe it for a year."

The most serious complication following angioplasty is a heart attack. That's why aggressive, state-of-the-art aftercare is an absolute must. Too many patients feel so well afterward that they stop taking their prescribed drugs. They're rudely awakened by a heart attack. They forget that their arteries were traumatized during the procedure and need months of healing.

Dr. Thomas Graboys elaborates: "Here's the paradox: You're doing a procedure to prevent heart attack but the person has a heart attack. It's part of reality, you just have to accept that. It gets down to maximizing medical therapy. All these patients should be on superaspirin, aggressive treatment of their cholesterol, aggressive treatment of their blood pressure, not smoking, the right kinds of vitamins such as folic acid to lower homocysteine levels. All of these are part of the new millennium of managing patients with coronary disease. It's totally different from the way it was ten or twenty years ago. That's an important point: We've made advances technically with these procedures, but we've also made tremendous advances in terms of medication."

BYPASS SURGERY

It's been around for more than a quarter of a century, but bypass surgery is truly new and improved with radically fewer deaths and much better immediate and long-term results. Just as important, there are many fewer complications such as stroke.

Still, this is an operation many of us have dreaded for years. The expectation is that your chest will be ripped open and that you'll have to spend weeks in the ICU recovering. Think again. Today's bypass surgery is a far gentler, safer, and better operation than it's ever been. Says Dr. Wayne Isom, "It's a million subtle little things that have changed. Better postoperative care,

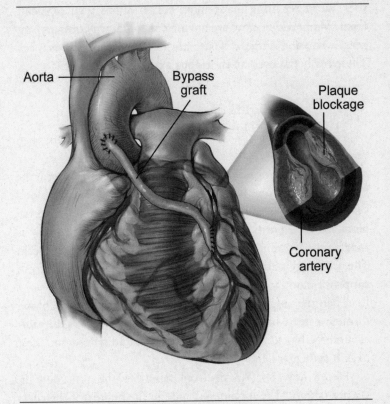

Aorta

Bypass graft

Plaque blockage

Coronary artery

better anesthetics. Ten years ago, people were spending ten days in the hospital after bypass surgery. Today many of these people are walking out of the hospital on the fourth day. Take valve repair. We're repairing many more valves rather than replacing them. Many people now are having the combined coronary surgery with valve surgery. These are huge therapeutic advances. There really has been an enormous amount of progress."

HOW THE STANDARD PROCEDURE IS DONE

First the surgeon isolates and prepares either a vein from the leg or an artery from the chest to be used as the bypassing blood vessel. The aim is to graft a vein as a conduit from above the blockage to a position below it—bypassing it. If an artery is used, its origin remains a major artery at the base of the neck. The other end is attached below the blockages to provide a fresh supply of blood from a vigorous artery.

Then the surgeon opens up your chest, reroutes the blood through a heart-lung machine, stops your heart, places the graft around the blockages, restarts your heart, and wires your chest back together.

Here's how Dr. Wayne Isom describes the procedure in greater detail: "The incision is made in the middle of the chest and it's spread apart gently and the heart is exposed. Then a new blood vessel, either an artery or a vein, is brought up and hooked up to the aorta. (It's like going around an obstruction in the Long Island Expressway—you take a side street. The expressway is the aorta, the side street is the graft and it goes around and back onto a highway, which is the coronary artery.)

"The heart is hooked up to the heart-lung machine and the heart and the lungs are completely bypassed so that there's no blood flow to the heart and lungs. The heart is stopped and is completely still and there is no blood in the vessels. To do this safely, you inject very cold solution into the heart. This stops the heart and almost eliminates completely any metabolism or oxygen consumption. So that allows you to work on the heart for a prolonged period of time, preferably an hour or less, but you can go three to four hours. And the machine itself is supplying the kidneys, the brain, the muscles, the liver, etc., with oxygen and nutrients."

CONSUMER QUESTION #7: DO YOU NEED THE OPERATION?

EXPERT ADVICE
Dr. Jeffrey Borer: "One reason to consider an operation is to prolong life. However, first, prolonging life is an alternative to not prolonging life, and the decision to undertake this strategy resides with the patient. Second, undertaking an operation for life prolongation requires that the potential for such benefit exists. The population in which life can be expected to be prolonged by bypass is pretty well circumscribed; it's not all that large. One reason for this is that, surprisingly to most people, medical therapy has advanced to the point where life expectancy is quite good for most patients with coronary artery disease without surgery. The people who actually are at greatest risk and who benefit to the greatest extent from bypass grafting are people with particularly severe disease, which usually means severe multivessel disease of various sorts."

Here are the key reasons to consider bypass surgery:

- Major blockages in all three main coronary arteries, particularly when associated with severe ischemia by noninvasive testing. In this case, the operation can extend life
  expectancy. At New York–Presbyterian Hospital, Weill
  Cornell Medical Center, of 800 coronary bypass procedures performed in a year, only 5 percent were performed
  on a single vessel. Most patients with single-vessel disease
  of a noncritical artery should consider medical or balloon
  therapy.
- A blockage in the left main coronary artery, which could
  cause sudden death or a massive heart attack.
- Any of the indications for balloon therapy, but balloon
  therapy is either not feasible or the risk is unacceptably
  high.
- Any of the indications for balloon therapy but you have
  diabetes.
- Multivessel disease involving the left anterior descending
  artery.
- Major blockage of the left main artery.
- Major blockage of any three arteries plus moderately
  weak pumping. (Dr. Jeffrey Moses counters that there are
  no data on nondiabetics to show that in this circumstance
  bypass is better than stenting.)
- Symptoms of coronary artery disease that interfere with
  day-to-day life and can't be controlled with medications
  or other procedures, such as balloon therapy. A great
  friend of mine and longtime marathon runner and cross-
  country skier experienced chest discomfort at very high
  exertional rates. An angiogram showed a 50 percent
  blockage of a coronary artery. He opted for surgery so
  that he could continue to lead his active lifestyle. A recent
  study in *Circulation* showed bypass surgery to be better
  than stent/angioplasty at relieving chest pain and improving quality of life in the year following the procedure.

There is another indication, says Dr. Wayne Isom: silent heart disease. "One of the things that cardiologists have found, and surgeons too, over the past thirty years, is that somewhere around 10 to 15 percent of the population do not have the normal pain patterns. They had a heart attack and never knew it, or they're on the treadmill doing a stress test and the stress test shows a major abnormality but they have no symptoms at all. So that's a group that you really have to consider. I've seen people who have terrible triple-vessel disease or even single-vessel disease who really need something done, and they don't have any symptoms at all."

He gives an example: "The patient I just operated on today had no symptoms at all. He's only sixty-one, very active, playing tennis, etc. He had a stress test that was positive, and it was not positive five years ago. He then had a thallium stress test (a radionuclide test that's noninvasive) that showed an abnormality of the heart. Then he went ahead and had a cardiac catheterization. Interestingly enough, he had no symptoms at all and his right coronary was nondominant, which means that he got all circulation from the left side. His left anterior descending, which is a critical vessel, sometime in the past closed off completely and he'd had a silent heart attack. He didn't know about it. The damage didn't show up on EKG, but it showed up on the catheterization. In addition, he had a 95 percent blockage of a branch off the circumflex artery. And off of that vessel had another 95 percent blockage. All this obstruction and no symptoms at all."

Dr. Isom adds to the list of candidates for bypass "people who are deemed inappropriate for medical therapy because of side effects or are so psychologically distraught that they just can't deal with it and want to go get 'fixed' and are willing to accept the risks as small as they are."

CONSUMER QUESTION #8: COULD YOUR OPERATION BE INAPPROPRIATE?

Here are the primary reasons a bypass operation may be considered inappropriate.

- You haven't exhausted drug therapy for symptom relief, and noninvasive testing suggests only a very modest foreseeable risk of heart attack or death. This is the number one reason for inappropriate balloon therapy or surgery. Patients have pain and want a quick fix. They press their doctors, who eventually give in. As safe as angioplasty and surgery are, this is an unnecessary risk.

- Blockages in your coronary arteries aren't severe enough to require surgery. If you've got decent blood flow through your arteries, you may not need surgery. Be sure to ask. Gung-ho surgeons may point out blockages on your angiogram, but they may not be significant in their location or severity. Dr. Wayne Isom says, "Bypass surgery is not appropriate if you don't have significant blockage; if the blockage is not above 50 to 60 percent, then you shouldn't operate. Make sure you get two opinions, since one surgeon might see 80 percent and another could counter, nope, just 50 percent. It's like looking at a painting."

    Dr. Jeffrey Moses adds that you should ask for a formal measurement to be certain of exactly how large the blockage is. "Wayne is referring here to what we call 'interobserver variability,' a very real phenomenon that is aggravated by the fact that most readings are made visually, with no objective measurements that might reduce error and variability. Also, there are highly sophisticated quantitative methods for assessing lesion severity, but these methods are not widely used clinically."

- Blockages in your arteries are too long or unwieldy to be

bypassed. There has to be a clean open section of blood vessel after the blockage to insert the new blood vessel. Otherwise bypass doesn't make sense. One reason the vessel may not be bypassable is that too many balloon therapies have been performed or stents implanted. Patients often make the mistake of postponing the inevitable. They get balloon therapies, which don't solve the problem but leave them unable to have bypass surgery.

- Chance of surviving surgery is poor. This conclusion may be based on the presence of other problems (diabetes, lung disease, kidney disease), or on evidence of severe prior heart muscle damage with associated valve abnormalities, or a combination of these or other factors. If your cardiologist or surgeon warns you that (who is obviously biased in favor of surgery) surgery is not right for you, take his or her word for it.
- Your blood vessel is blocked, but a new blood supply has emerged that takes its place. This is called neovascularization, and it means that many small blood vessels have grown around the blockages to supply the heart muscle. Says Dr. Wayne Isom, "Bypass is not appropriate if, for example, there is one vessel involved that's completely obstructed but it's collateralized, it's done what I call an internal bypass." "That is, unless it is causing symptoms or a major disturbance of blood flow," adds Dr. Jeffrey Moses.

EXCEPTIONS

Surgeons like Dr. Lawrence Cohn bristle at the accusation of too much inappropriate surgery. Dr. Cohn, whom I've sent my own mother to, is most concerned about the hundreds of thousands of patients who die of a heart attack every year without risk ever being detected.

"There are people who have absolutely no chest pain and they're fine, and then all of a sudden they drop dead. Well, it turns out that unless you do an angiogram of some of these people with positive exercise testing, you may never know what's going on. So if someone were to make that claim, after an angiogram, I'd accept the criticism. But if you don't do an angiogram on the patients, you don't know what you have.

"Take Jim Fixx, the runner. He did the diet and exercise yet still dropped dead of a heart attack. He had an undiagnosed coronary artery lesion. See, what I'm saying is, it's a complicated business. The study of the coronary arteries with an angiogram is I think quite important. And it's becoming increasingly important and becoming increasingly safer to do, by the way."

I keep reminding you of the missing half, those whose first symptom of heart disease is a heart attack or sudden death. Dr. Cohn is concerned that the current guidelines could allow those with silent heart disease to slip through the cracks.

"Sometimes people have blockages and no symptoms. That's a very dangerous group, because those are the ones who can die suddenly. So if you're a vigorous person, if you have a family history, if you have a genetic influence, if you've had a bad diet, if you've smoked—those kind of people probably ought to get a specialist's opinion and an exercise screening test. It's a very excellent way to pick out the people who don't have symptoms but still have very severe coronary disease and could drop dead."

CONSUMER QUESTION #9: HOW DO YOU PICK A HOSPITAL?

The prospect of bypass surgery used to put fear into hearts of patients. Yet now it is one of the safest operations you can have—if you're in the right hands. As techniques and equipment have improved, the number of serious complications has dropped dramatically. There are, however, still serious risks, including stroke, heart attack, and death, especially if you are a high-risk patient or in the wrong hands. This is why it's critical to be in the very best hospital with the very best doctors. Even as a high-risk patient, your chances of failure can be cut sharply.

VOLUME

Study after study has shown that those centers performing the most procedures have the best outcome. Practice really does make perfect. Give yourself the best possible opportunity not just to survive but to thrive by choosing the right center.

This is where consumer medicine has hit its peak, since it's easy for untrained patients to choose centers based on a small number of criteria. High-volume centers concentrate on the expertise of an entire team, from the bypass technicians and anesthesiologists to the ICU nurses. Studies have shown that excellent surgeons can get poor results when the team doesn't match up. One approach is to go to nationally recognized centers of excellence such as Mass General in Boston, New York–Presbyterian Hospital, or the Cleveland Clinic. However, if you want or need to stay local, consider the report card below.

Critics say that a high-volume hospital is necessary only for patients at high risk. A recent study from the Veterans Affairs Outcomes Group in the Department of Veteran Affairs Medical Center in White River Junction, Vermont, found that the greatest volume-related differences in mortality did occur in patients at highest risk, but they also found volume-related differences in lower-risk patients. The researchers concluded, "Although the merits of volume-based referral initiatives can be debated on many grounds, there seems to be little rationale for restricting these initiatives to high-risk patients." A number of medical groups have established criteria for the minimum annual number of open-heart surgeries considered necessary for a hospital to maintain proficiency, ranging from the American College of Surgeon's 150 operations a year to the American College of Cardiology's 300 operations to the Society of Thoracic Surgeons institutional minimum of 500.

Despite the differences in these standards, one thing is consistent: The number of deaths rises as the hospital's annual frequency of surgery falls. And it is falling all over, as angioplasty increases, so last year's numbers may not be relevant this year. You should know the number of bypass operations performed each year at the hospitals you are considering for your surgery. Although bypass surgery can be a routine operation, you can run an extraordinarily and unnecessarily high risk of complications or death at the wrong hospital.

DEATH RATE

This is the most important and easiest consumer rating number to obtain. Says Harvard's Lawrence Cohn, "Right now, the mortality rate for the uncomplicated coronary bypass procedure should be no higher than 2 percent no matter how few you do. If you're in a hospital for an uncomplicated coronary bypass procedure that's not achieving an operative mortality of 1 to 2 percent, you'd better get your coat and hat on and get the heck out of there as fast as you can. If the hospital is doing a large number of reoperations or operating on cardiogenic shock or emergencies, the rate may be higher than that." Dr. Cohn's institution, the Brigham and Women's Hospital, has a risk-adjusted death rate of 1 percent.

Look too for a low complication rate.

REPORT CARDS

How do you find these data? It's on report cards. States like New York issue their own very successful report cards each year. Medicare has one of the most comprehensive sets of data. Magazines such as *U.S. News & World Report* issue rankings of hospitals.

Dr. Wayne Isom says, "*U.S. News & World Report* is pretty good, but there is some discrepancy there. If you want to use their list of places, I would say with the top twenty you wouldn't go wrong. I wouldn't try to say that number three is better than number twenty, though. This gives you a ballpark idea."

One major drawback of the report card system is that doctors, just like anyone else, don't want a bad report card. That means many hesitate to operate on very high-risk cases and ruin their score. The flip side is that if they have agreed to operate on you, you've got a pretty decent chance of success. Some surgeons with poorer numbers say that the tables don't reflect the high-risk cases they do take. That can be true. However, doctors at New York–Presbyterian Hospital, Weill Cornell Center operate on very sick high-risk patients, and the hospital still gets the highest marks with the lowest mortality rates. Be careful of hospital-generated report cards. Says Dr. Wayne Isom, "Be careful about the hospital self-reporting results, because the hospital is not going to put its bad results up. If it's hospital generated, that means it's generated by the advertising firm employed by the hospital."

RISK-FACTOR ADJUSTMENT

Wayne Isom says, "Consider a forty-five-year-old athlete who's never had a heart attack and has a left main stem blockage that is life-threatening. His risk is going to be way less than

1 percent. If that person's eighty years old and he's had three heart attacks and his heart muscle is very weakened and he's in the middle of a heart attack when you operate on him and perform a quadruple bypass, his risk may be 25 to 30 percent."

There is another risk to consider, the risk of not having an operation that might save your life. Dr. Wayne Isom explains: "Many patients and their doctors opt for the quick fix. Since bypass can be dangerous, the experts would rather you vigorously pursue medical treatment before you consider surgery. Well, sometimes the medical treatment is more dangerous than the surgical procedure. The risk in an open-heart or coronary bypass procedure, if it's done electively and not in the face of a reoperation or a major heart attack, is less than 1 percent. If you've got, let's say, three vessels involved, even though you're not symptomatic, your risk of dying [on drug therapy alone] is at least that much, maybe more, for each year. So surgery might be less risky."

THE TEAM

It's also not just the surgeon; it's the team and how long the team has been there. Wayne Isom continues, "You want to ask questions about cardiac anesthesia. What's the staffing in the ICU? Is it an academic center? One of the reasons I say an academic center is that some people say they don't want interns and residents experimenting on them, but if you go to a place where there are interns and residents, you've got someone looking over their shoulder constantly. So if I tried to do some unnecessary procedure, there would be two or three people saying, 'Hey, wait a minute, you can't do that, there's not an indication for that.' Another analogy is you can have the best pilot in the world to fly you from here to Los Angeles, but if you don't have a copilot, someone checking the gas, the radio, a navigator, someone making sure the jet is working fine, you don't want to fly with him.

You also want to know how long the team has been together as a team. You could recruit a terrific staff to a new program and have poor results until they are molded into a team."

· There are hospitals across the country that have risk factors of 1 percent or less due not just to the experience of the surgeons but also to improved surgical techniques, improved materials, and improved post-op techniques.

QUALITY OF THE POST-OP TEAM

Most deaths do not occur in the operating room. After your surgery, cardiologists should be readily available, twenty-four hours a day, in a fully staffed and certified cardiac care unit. They are the specialists best qualified to treat potentially fatal irregular heart rhythms. You should also look for programs with a full-time thoracic surgery training program. If you develop complications at four A.M., you want a surgeon familiar with your case to be available.

THE REPORT CARD

HealthGrades has allowed me to publish its 2004 list of five-star hospitals for bypass surgery. HealthGrades methods are described in the section on balloon therapy, pages 219–20.

ALABAMA
University of Alabama Hospital, Birmingham
Riverview Regional Medical Center, Gadsden

ARIZONA
Arizona Heart Hospital, Phoenix
Walter O. Boswell Memorial Hospital, Sun City
Northwest Medical Center, Tucson
Tucson Heart Hospital, Tucson

ARKANSAS
St. Joseph's Mercy Health Center, Hot Springs

CALIFORNIA
Methodist Hospital of Southern California, Arcadia
Grossmont Hospital, La Mesa
St. John's Regional Medical Center, Oxnard
Mercy General Hospital, Sacramento
Marian Medical Center, Santa Maria
San Ramon Regional Medical Center, San Ramon

COLORADO
Memorial Hospital, Colorado Springs
Centura Health Porter Adventist Hospital, Denver

CONNECTICUT
Yale New Haven Hospital, New Haven

FLORIDA
Morton Plant Hospital, Clearwater
Holmes Regional Medical Center, Melbourne
Munroe Regional Medical Center, Ocala
Leesburg Regional Medical Center, Leesburg
Central Florida Regional Hospital, Sanford
Delray Medical Center, Delray Beach

ILLINOIS
Northwest Community Hospital, Arlington Heights
St. John's Hospital, Springfield
Carle Foundation Hospital, Urbana
Central Dupage Hospital, Winfield
St. Francis Hospital and Health Center, Blue Island
Riverside Medical Center, Kankakee
St. Elizabeth Hospital, Belleville

Advocate Christ Medical Center, Oak Lawn
Advocate Lutheran General Hospital, Park Ridge
Alexian Brothers Medical Center, Elk Grove Village

INDIANA
Elkhart General Hospital, Elkhart
Memorial Hospital, South Bend
Saint Joseph's Regional Medical Center, South Bend
Methodist Hospital Southlake, Merrillville

IOWA
Mercy Medical Center North Iowa, Mason City

KANSAS
Kansas Heart Hospital, Wichita

KENTUCKY
The Medical Center, Bowling Green

LOUISIANA
Southwest Medical Center, Lafayette

MAINE
Maine Medical Center, Portland

MARYLAND
Union Memorial Hospital, Baltimore
Sacred Heart Hospital, Cumberland

MASSACHUSETTS
Brigham and Women's Hospital, Boston
New England Medical Center, Boston
UMass Memorial Medical Center, Worcester

MICHIGAN
University of Michigan Health System, Ann Arbor
Oakwood Hospital and Medical Center, Dearborn
Northern Michigan Hospital, Petoskey
St. Joseph Mercy Oakland, Pontiac
Spectrum Health Downtown Campus, Grand Rapids
Munson Medical Center, Traverse City
William Beaumont Hospital, Royal Oak
St. John Hospital and Medical Center, Detroit
Genesys Regional Medical Center, Grand Blanc

MINNESOTA
St. Luke's Hospital, Duluth
Abbott Northwestern Hospital, Minneapolis
Hennepin County Medical Center, Minneapolis
St. Cloud Hospital, Saint Cloud

MISSOURI
St. Joseph Health Center, Kansas City

MONTANA
St. Vincent Healthcare, Billings

NEW HAMPSHIRE
Portsmouth Regional Hospital, Portsmouth

NEW JERSEY
Morristown Memorial Hospital, Morristown
St. Francis Medical Center, Trenton
Jersey Shore University Medical Center, Neptune
St. Barnabas Medical Center, Livingston

NEW MEXICO
Memorial Medical Center, Las Cruces

NEW YORK
St. Peter's Hospital, Albany
Lenox Hill Hospital, New York City
Rochester General Hospital, Rochester
Staten Island University Hospital, Staten Island
New York Hospital Medical Center of Queens,
    Flushing
Montefiore Medical Center, Bronx
St. Joseph's Hospital Health Center, Syracuse
Winthrop University Hospital, Mineola
St. Francis Hospital, Roslyn
Long Island Jewish Medical Center, New Hyde Park

NORTH CAROLINA
Duke University Hospital, Durham
Moses H. Cone Memorial Hospital & Women's Hospital,
    Greensboro

NORTH DAKOTA
Meritcare Hospital, Fargo

OHIO
Toledo Hospital, Toledo
EMH Regional Medical Center, Elyria
Cleveland Clinic Foundation, Cleveland
Metro Valley Hospital, Cleveland
Aultman Hospital, Canton
Miami Valley Hospital, Dayton
Parma Community General Hospital, Parma

OREGON
Sacred Heart Medical Center, Eugene
Rogue Valley Medical Center, Medford

PENNSYLVANIA
Saint Vincent Health System, Erie
Hamot Medical Center, Erie
Frankford Hospital, Philadelphia
St. Luke's Hospital, Bethlehem
Lancaster General Hospital, Lancaster
Lehigh Valley Hospital, Allentown
York Hospital, York
Butler Memorial Hospital, Butler
Mercy Hospital, Scranton
St. Clair Memorial Hospital, Pittsburgh

RHODE ISLAND
Miriam Hospital, Providence

SOUTH CAROLINA
Grand Strand Regional Medical Center,
    Myrtle Beach

TENNESSEE
St. Thomas Hospital, Nashville
University of Tennessee Memorial Hospital,
    Knoxville

TEXAS
Christus Santa Rosa Hospital, San Antonio
Conroe Regional Medical Center, Conroe
McAllen Medical Center, McAllen
Nacogdoches Medical Center, Nacogdoches
College Station Medical Center, College Station

UTAH
McKay Dee Hospital Center, Ogden
St. Mark's Hospital, Salt Lake City

VIRGINIA
Sentara Norfolk General Hospital, Norfolk
Virginia Baptist Hospital and Lynchburg General,
    Lynchburg
Inova Alexandria Hospital, Alexandria
Lewis-Gale Medical Center, Salem
Sentara Virginia Beach General Hospital, Virginia Beach
Bon Secours St. Mary's Hospital, Richmond
CJW Medical Center, Richmond
Henrico Doctors' Hospital Forest Campus/Parham
    Campus, Richmond

WYOMING
Wyoming Medical Center, Casper

Missing are some of the biggest big-name hospitals, such as Harvard's Massachusetts's General and New York Hospital, hospitals I can personally vouch for. Dr. Wayne Isom recommends the top twenty on the *U.S. News & World Report* list.

See my advice on page 224 for what to do if you need bypass surgery and none of the above hospitals is near you.

CONSUMER QUESTION #10: HOW DO YOU CHOOSE A SURGEON?

Mickey Mantle had great stats and so should your surgeon. Cardiac surgeons have real, hard numbers, which help you decide who is best. These numbers show death rate and complications.

First and foremost, your surgeon should do a large number of procedures. How many? Dr. Lawrence Cohn has done 5,000 and continues to do 100 a year. These do not all need to be bypass surgeries, since great open heart surgeons also operate on heart valves and perform other, more complicated procedures. Wayne Isom counsels, "I think a surgeon needs to be doing at least 100 open-heart surgeries a year, not necessarily 100 bypasses. You want to be careful that more is not necessarily better. One surgeon may do 300 simple bypass surgeries in low-risk patients whereas Larry or Wayne may do 100 very complex patients with severe disease."

When you pick a surgeon, you're also picking the team he or she operates with. For that reason, take a close look at the hospital and perhaps choose that first. There are surgeons whose reputations are bigger than the hospitals at which they operate. In the past, they were the legendary De Bakey and Cooley. Today they are Cosgrove at the Cleveland Clinic, Isom at Weill Cornell Medical Center, Cohn at Brigham and Women's, Quinn at Maine Medical Center, and others. Still, for the surgeon to have excellent results, the institution must maintain a high standard of quality.

There are some basic formalities, such as credentialing by the American Board of Thoracic Surgery, but it is highly unlikely that a surgeon at a major center isn't spectacularly well credentialed. Where the rubber meets the road is really the surgeon's experience and outcome.

Says Lawrence Cohn, "I had a guy yesterday ask me how many bypasses had I done, because it's the only time he's going to have one.

"So I said I'd done 5,000 bypass operations myself. "So he said, 'okay, how many do you do a year?' He sounded like he was reading your book!

"And I said, 'Well, a whole unit does about 800 cases a year of bypass and I myself probably do 100.' "

One hundred a year is a good round number to look for. The real bottom line is the outcome. The risks of the operations depend on each patient. But overall the death rate should be no higher than 2 percent. For low-risk surgery, the death rate should be less than 1 percent.

This is the dawn of the consumer era in medicine. Cars, computers, and financial services are all incredibly complicated, yet they have been reduced to simple buying choices by consumerism.

In all of medicine, bypass surgery comes the closest to attaining that ideal for the ease with which the consumer can make a pretty good choice. Just as consumerism improved cars, computers, and financial services, it dramatically improved surgical results as well. When reports were first published about ten years ago, death rates were over 7 percent at some institutions in New York State. Now most hospitals have death rates closer to 2 percent. I interviewed a surgeon at St. Peter's Hospital in Albany who was the lowest-rated surgeon in New York State. It turned out that he was extremely well trained. But he got burned by procedures at his hospital, which rushed patients into surgery too quickly. As the low man on the totem pole, he got most of the emergency cases. Patient preparation and the team around him rapidly improved. On the HealthGrades list, St. Peter's now ranks as a five-star hospital. The report card system helped point out the problems and help this hospital and others improve.

VEIN OR ARTERY?

Dr. Lawrence Cohn advises, "Nowadays, in 99.9 percent of the cases, an artery that's taken from the chest is absolutely standard. It's called internal mammary to left anterior descending bypass. It should be understood absolutely from the get-go that that is part of the operation."

If you are going to have your left anterior descending artery bypassed, you definitely want an artery used. Since blockage of this artery can kill you, you want a graft that has the best chance of remaining open, and that's an artery. If you've had a previous operation or bypass surgery, the artery may be too badly scarred or damaged to use. Younger patients should also opt for an arterial bypass, since they want the benefits of their operation to last longer.

WHAT TO EXPECT AFTER CORONARY BYPASS SURGERY

The care of your new bypass grafts goes a long way to preserving them for years and even decades. Take these measures seriously.

The journal *Circulation* provides a simple A, B, C, D, E, F checklist.

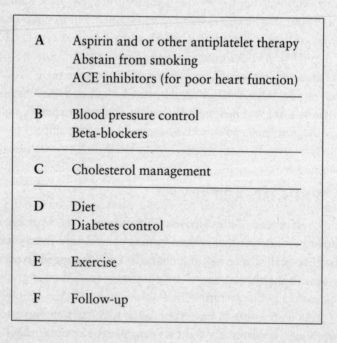

A	Aspirin and or other antiplatelet therapy Abstain from smoking ACE inhibitors (for poor heart function)
B	Blood pressure control Beta-blockers
C	Cholesterol management
D	Diet Diabetes control
E	Exercise
F	Follow-up

Be sure to discuss each item on the list with your doctors. Remember that bypass surgery does not change the underlying disease process, which is relentless. That's why drug therapy is so critically important.

CUTTING-EDGE BYPASS SURGERY

Many top surgeons, such as Wayne Isom, still believe strongly in the standard bypass surgery because of the tremendous precision that is possible in sewing the actual vessels together. Still, there has been a great deal of buzz about new surgeries, from minimally invasive to keyhole. Of these, there are two that have survived: off-bypass and robotic.

OFF-BYPASS

Some neurologists have been fearful that patients on a heart-lung machine may suffer subtle neurological damage. Patients who are older or have borderline kidney or lung function are at highest risk of complications on the heart-lung machine.

To try and reduce these neurological microinjuries and make bypass less physiologically stressful to older or sicker patients, a minimally invasive surgery, known as MIDCAB, is performed while the heart is still beating. The surgeon creates small holes in the chest to insert instruments and makes a small incision directly over the clogged coronary artery. An artery from inside the chest wall is detached and connected to the clogged artery to bypass the occlusion.

Don't opt for this technique unless the team does hundreds of these each year and has great results. It's good for only one or possibly two vessels. This is a very technically challenging operation for only those surgeons with great skill. In New York State, its use has decreased from 5 percent to less than 1 percent. Many experts say that some degree of precision is lost.

Dr. Jeffrey Borer says, "It is true that some people can have a problem with the heart-lung machine. Most of these are very elderly, and most have very severe atherosclerosis. Yet people should not be scared about being on the heart-lung machine. Recent data from a study at New York–Presbyterian Cornell indicate that the subtle neurological problems that have been associated with the heart-lung machine are largely attributable to use of inadequate perfusion pressure [the blood pressure generated by the machine] during the procedure. When higher perfusion pressures are used, the neurological problems largely disappear. Having said that, however, if you could do the job without adding that dimension, that would be fine." My own mother did very well on the heart-lung at age ninety by having high perfusion pressure.

The American Heart Association has been carefully monitoring these procedures. Although MIDCAB seems to be easier on the patient and less expensive than open-heart bypass, there may be complications that require the chest to be opened.

All in all, if you're too sick for traditional bypass and need a single-vessel bypass to extend your life, this may be a great option. But listen to Dr. Wayne Isom, who performs bypasses almost every day. Off-bypass requires a lot of precision. "You have to get all the vessels that are involved and you also have to do an A+ connection. The vessels are smaller than a pencil lead, about 1.5 mm, and the suture that you're using is about as big as your hair. The accuracy that it takes to do an A+ connection, well, imagine that you took the eye of a sewing needle and decreased it by three-quarters. If you're on-bypass, you stop the heart, it's completely still, there's no blood in it. You can thread the needle ten out of ten times. Now if you're off-bypass, the heart is still beating because you're not supporting the circulation at all, there's still a little blood coming out. If you move that needle up and down a little bit and throw a little blood on it periodically, you can probably, with a little practice, thread that needle six out of ten times. And initially that would look okay. Maybe you would be able to get out of the hospital in three days if we do it that way. But if you're back in three years, we haven't done you any favors."

Beware too that surgeons like Wayne Isom see this as a marketing tool so that a hospital can say it does the minimally invasive technique, when it actually depends on the individual case. Certain centers in New York "really push this thing to get people to come but then still end up doing the open-heart surgery because it's indicated. There are a lot of places using that as a marketing tool. They use that to get you there, then they'll say, 'Oh, we'll try to do it that way but we may have to make a decision when we get there.' I've heard of patients coming to a hospital for three or four bypasses and they are told, 'We think we'll do this through a small incision.' Then they're put to sleep and opened up, and the surgeon does all the bypasses the normal way. He says, 'Oh we couldn't do it, it was too difficult.' So be careful about that."

Dr. Isom is also concerned that the neurological damage from traditional bypass surgery may be exaggerated. He operated on David Letterman. "Letterman even says his thinking is better, he was on the pump nearly two hours, and if your memory and timing are better, it's hard to postulate that there is damage. If you were causing strokes, a guy like this who was on the heart-lung machine quite a while would be at the greatest risk."

He says that the concern goes back to a study that was done in the 1990s at Duke University. It showed a loss of cognitive function over years after being on the heart-lung machine. Trouble with the study was that it was a single-institution study; it was done in the early 1990s and techniques now are fifteen years better; and there was no control group ("amazing it was even published," he says).

The bottom line is that if your doctor and his or her team are excellent, and you are at a first-rate hospital, the risk of on-bypass is very low. And new research indicates that the chances of having to return for more surgery or another procedure may be higher with off-bypass than on-bypass.

ROBOTIC-ASSISTED CORONARY BYPASS SURGERY

First, the surgeon makes two tiny incisions so the robot can insert its arms into your chest. The robot then strips a key artery from the chest wall to be used as the bypass graft. Under the left breast, the surgeon makes a very small, keyhole-like incision through which the actual bypass is performed. Says Dr. Lawrence Cohn, "You can do a terrific bypass that way. But that's mainly for one or two vessels, not really for the whole big thing that most people have. That's the only so-called keyhole surgery we are doing now. Eventually you will be able to do a robotic-assisted bypass without opening the chest at all, but that's a little bit away."

Since this is performed on one or two vessels, surgeons are competing with cardiologists for the cases. The cardiologists often win. Furthermore, this is still considered experimental.

The original procedure, says Dr. Cohn, is no longer performed. "The keyhole way that was done ten years ago has been completely discredited, it doesn't work." Wayne Isom echoes, "The minimally invasive keyhole surgery that was popular five or six years ago is rarely done now."

CHOOSING BETWEEN BALLOON THERAPY AND BYPASS SURGERY

Angioplasty in many cases today replaces the need for bypass surgery. Cardiologists agree with surgeons that at least 20 percent of patients requiring a procedure would benefit from surgery. Surgeons agree that at least 20 percent of patients requiring a procedure would benefit from angioplasty. But that leaves a huge gray area in between. It is an enormous battleground with both surgeons and cardiologists vying for patients. Cardiologists are carving out a bigger and bigger piece of the pie for themselves. You want to be certain that you don't undergo unnecessary surgery when balloon therapy would have worked. Alternatively, you want to be very wary of getting caught in this battleground, having a highly experimental and potentially dangerous balloon therapy procedure. In the end, you are likely to end up a winner. Both of these procedures are far safer today than ever before.

Now that you've read through these two sections, you may still not be sure which procedure is best for you. Here are two good pieces of advice from the experts.

EXPERT ADVICE

Dr. Steven Nissen: "Good people are going to agree most of the time but not all the time. And so there are shades of gray. Depending on which hospital will do the procedure may make a really big difference.

"Let's suppose you're at hospital A, which has exceptionally good surgery and somewhat weaker interventional cardiology. That's a place where surgery is good and angioplasty is weak, so you're probably better off having an operation. There are other places where surgery is not as strong and where the interventional people are particularly skilled."

EXPERT ADVICE

Dr. Wayne Isom: "I think if a patient needs to have something done, and the indications for surgery and angioplasty are about the same, it's worth trying an angioplasty with a stent maybe once. But the problem is when a patient keeps coming back and gets more stents put in. When bypass surgery works, it can work exceptionally well. Look at someone like Larry King. He says, 'Over sixteen years post-op from a quintuple and I've done seventy-five hundred shows since then.' And he says he's got two young sons, 'all without Viagra.' "

So how do you decide? Go to a major university center that has an excellent reputation for both surgery and balloon therapy and where there is no economic incentive to perform one procedure rather than the other.

OTHER MEDICAL DEVICES

IMPLANTABLE DEFIBRILLATORS

Defibrillators (so-called pacemakers) used to be big bulky boxes the size of a lunch pail that paramedics rushed to a patient with cardiac arrest. Breakthrough companies like Medtronics have designed miniature defibrillators that can be implanted in your chest. Dick Cheney has one. But there is now a new revolution in their use. Anyone with a weak or bad heart can benefit from having a defibrillator implanted, not just those with a previously diagnosed problem with their heart's electrical system. This is the key way to prevent most sudden death from an electrical disturbance in the heart, which is what a defibrillator is designed to prevent.

The latest implantable cardiodefibrillator (ICD) is about the size of a small cell phone. It is two devices in one. First, it acts as a pacemaker that can sense an abnormally slow heartbeat and then supply the missing beats to get your heart rate back to normal. Second, it is a cardioverter, which senses an abnormally rapid heart rate and then supplies a large jolt of electricity to restore a normal heart rhythm. A recent study of 1,200 people showed that implanting an ICD resulted in 30 percent fewer deaths.

Patients with weak heart muscle or severe disturbances of the heart's electrical rhythm who are prone to sudden cardiac arrest should consider having a defibrillator implanted in their chest. The key is that most patients in heart failure or with low ejection fractions are not considered, and they should be. My father had a weakened heart and long-standing electrical disturbances in his heart. He was considered for a pacemaker, but his doctors never followed through.

EXPERT ADVICE

Dr. Jeffrey Moses: "We found out that anybody who has a bad heart could use [a defibrillator]. In one study, patients who just have a weak heart and coronary disease do better with a defibrillator. That's a big issue because there are hundreds of thousands of people with weak hearts in this country who qualify, and if everyone got one, that would add about $50 billion to the health bill. So we're still struggling with that one.

"It's clear that the broader applications of defibrillators to a much wider group of patients, not just what used to be sudden death survivors, is a very important advantage. Like Dick Cheney. He didn't drop dead, he didn't have a lethal arrhythmia; he had some abnormal beats. They put this in to prevent him from dropping dead. Cheney is a prime example of what was done in that regard."

ARTIFICIAL HEARTS

LEFT VENTRICULAR ASSIST DEVICES (LVADS)

It was 1996. I stood with the legendary Michael De Bakey in Berlin at the German Heart Institute. History was about to be made. A young German man lay near death on the operating table. As doctors opened his chest, we peered over to see a heart that was almost black. In just minutes, a new device was implanted in his chest. It was the size of just two double A batteries. The De Bakey heart began to spin at ten thousand revolutions per minute. The patient's heart miraculously changed from black to pink and began to pump with vigor. That day was the beginning of a new age when, even with the worst heart disease, there would be hope with cheap, easily available artificial hearts.

Today mechanical devices offer remarkable hope to hundreds of thousands of heart patients. Best of all, the De Bakey device can pull lives back from the grasp of the grim reaper. The great news is that 95 percent of people with severe heart disease don't need a whole artificial heart but can survive and thrive with this small precision jewel, instead of lugging around something the size of a small washer-drier. The De Bakey heart has other applications as well. Patients with heart failure can literally give their hearts a rest with the temporary implantation of the De Bakey heart. Robert Jarvik has also pioneered a new LVAD, as have others.

Left ventricular assist devices have recently been approved by the Food and Drug Administration to support the circulation of patients with end-stage heart failure awaiting cardiac transplantation. The hope is that an LVAD may give their heart a chance to recover on its own. The Randomized Evaluation of Mechanical Assistance for the Treatment of Congestive Heart Failure (REMATCH) trial is a multicenter study supported by the National Heart, Lung, and Blood Institute to compare long-term implantation of left ventricular assist devices with optimal medical management for patients with end-stage heart failure who require, but do not qualify to receive, cardiac transplantation. In the long term, it's hoped that miniature LVADs will work as permanently implanted devices. Since 90 percent of heart transplants are performed for left heart failure, in theory an LVAD could takes its place. In theory, if you have a massive heart attack, doctors could implant one of these devices.

If you or a family member is in a hospital from seemingly irreversible heart failure with a grim prognosis, raise the idea of an LVAD. My own experience is that you should start asking at the beginning of the downhill slope when the operation has a better chance of success. You may be rebuffed, but it can't hurt to ask about institutions that offer this device. Also, if you are an older patient with heart failure who is not a candidate for transplant, be sure to ask about the REMATCH trial and the availability of LVADs.

ON THE HORIZON

ABIOCOR

For those few individuals who suffer the failure of the whole heart, instead of the more vulnerable left heart, there is a remarkable new artificial heart. I was able to see one of the first prototypes of the Abiocor heart, which has overcome some problems of the earlier Louisville heart. The breakthrough is the creation of materials that line the inner surfaces of the artificial heart to prevent blood clots, which cause stroke, the fatal flaw of previous artificial hearts. This is the holy grail of cardiac devices, and efforts are ongoing to try to bring it to market.

ANGIOGENESIS

The wild West of cardiology is gene therapy. Specially selected genes are ingeniously implanted into thickly clogged arteries in the sickest of hearts. These genes encourage hearts to "grow" their own new blood vessels. Imagine a patient who is too sick for bypass surgery or whose arteries are all but slammed shut, making balloon therapy impossible. The hope for the future is to avoid surgery altogether. In the here and now, heart bypass patients are treated with a timed-release capsule of a substance that promotes the growth of new blood vessels during surgery.

STEM CELLS

A recent issue of *Circulation* showed that injecting a patient's own cells into a coronary artery several days after a heart attack "speeds the healing process and strengthens the heart's pumping power."

Good, solid decision making based on hard facts and figures is the key to selecting a procedure that will work well for you. Even in the heat of a crisis, take the time to briefly review the key points in this chapter to be sure that the procedure is appropriate and that you are at an institution that has a published record of excellent results. A friend of our family's was scheduled to have valve surgery. The hospital performing the procedure did not have a first-rate track record. I tried to convince the family the evening before that this was a bad decision. The family said it was too late to change hospitals, even though it was an elective procedure. I told the family it was not too late until the chest was open. They stuck by their guns. The patient suffered a debilitating stroke from which he never recovered.

The right procedures for the right patient are some of the greatest miracles in modern medicine. If you simply make certain that your procedure is appropriate for your condition and use the simple consumer approach to selecting the right team, you stand an excellent chance of coming through with a great result. Many of the missing half I have tracked through this book would never have suffered a heart attack or died if they had had the right procedure.

You and I are at the dawn of a revolution in which our children and grandchildren may never suffer from coronary artery disease. Chances are excellent that you will benefit from much of this revolution if you follow the seven steps set forth in this book. You may be able to slow, stop, or even reverse whatever narrowing you have in your coronary arteries. Having read this book puts you in front of 99 percent of those who have heart disease or are at risk for it.

Cardiology has, however, lost much of the glamour it had a decade ago in the news media. As a result, there is much less excitement and a great deal more complacency about heart disease than ever before. The fear factor about heart disease has largely evaporated. Yet you've seen the numbers, and they are staggering. Fifty percent of men and 63 percent of women who die suddenly of coronary artery disease have no previous symptoms. This missing half of heart patients die before they ever reach the hospital. Many fail to follow even a single step in this book. But you now have the core knowledge on which to build a first-rate lifesaving plan.

I offer you my congratulations for taking the time and effort to master these concepts. In the end, saving your life and that of someone you love is easy. You need to know only the most basic principles to radically improve your chances. By eliminating your risk of heart disease, still the number one cause of death in America, you have vastly increased your chances of living a robust life to a great old age.

APPENDIX

BODY MASS INDEX

Being overweight or obese is defined as having a Body Mass Index of 25 or higher. You can calculate your Body Mass Index by using this mathematical formula:

$$\text{B.M.I.} = \left(\frac{\text{WEIGHT IN POUNDS}}{(\text{HEIGHT IN INCHES}) \times (\text{HEIGHT IN INCHES})} \right) \times 703$$

Then apply the result to this chart.

Less than 18.5	18.5–24.9	25–29.9	30–39.9	40 or higher
UNDERWEIGHT	NORMAL	OVERWEIGHT	OBESE	EXTREMELY OBESE

For those who lack good math skills, simply draw lines from your height on the left and weight below and see where they meet. For example, someone 5 foot 8 and 145 pounds (dark horizontal and vertical lines) is at a normal weight. B.M.I. applies to men and women twenty years of age or older.

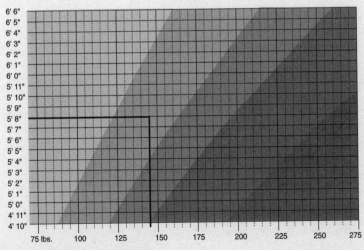

Source: Centers for Disease Control and Prevention

INDEX

263

Index

Index

Index